When the Drugs Don't Work

When the Drugs Don't Work

The Hidden Pandemic That Could End Modern Medicine

Anirban Mahapatra

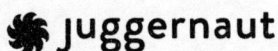

JUGGERNAUT BOOKS
C-I-128, First Floor, Sangam Vihar, Near Holi Chowk,
New Delhi 110080, India

First published by Juggernaut Books 2024

Copyright © Anirban Mahapatra 2024

10 9 8 7 6 5 4 3 2 1

P-ISBN: 9789353459093
E-ISBN: 9789353453817

The views and opinions expressed in this book are the author's own. The facts contained herein were reported to be true as on the date of publication by the author to the publishers of the book, and the publishers are not in any way liable for their accuracy or veracity.

All rights reserved. No part of this publication may be reproduced, transmitted, or stored in a retrieval system in any form or by any means without the written permission of the publisher.

Typeset in Adobe Caslon Pro by R. Ajith Kumar, Noida

Printed at Nutech Print Services - India

For Rituparna, whose unwavering support makes all things possible

Contents

Preface   ix

1. A Daily Tragedy   1
2. Superbug Signatures   19
3. Blindness in a Bottle   29
4. The New Delhi Story   47
5. The Last Line Falls   71
6. The Eye of the Storm   81
7. The World Outside   95
8. The World Within Us   115
9. How We Stumbled on Antibiotics (and Resistance)   129
10. Drowning in Antibiotics   157
11. Fat Animals and Antibiotics   171
12. A Market Failure   179
13. The Next Generation   195

Contents

14. Beyond Antibiotics   207
15. The Hidden Pandemic   231

Additional Resources   239
Notes   241
Acknowledgements   263

Preface
What This Book Is About

In recent years, there have been several books written about the rise of bacteria that can't be treated with common antibiotics for scientists, physicians, economists, historians, and policymakers. This, however, is not one of them.

This book has been written to raise awareness of a health crisis that affects you, me, and everyone else. The idea came from a frank disclosure made by a family member, someone who had a nightmare encounter with superbugs – a bacterial infection that did not respond to antibiotics.

Perhaps you know someone who has faced a similar crisis. A premature newborn confined to an intensive care unit (ICU) struggling for life with a superbug infection. Or a urinary tract infection that just wouldn't go away. Maybe a routine surgical procedure or a Caesarean section that led to a prolonged stay in a hospital.

If you live in India, Bangladesh, Pakistan, or a similarly

populous and dense country where antibiotics are readily accessible, it's highly likely you've directly encountered a superbug or know someone who has faced this threat. The rapid spread of antibiotic-resistant bacteria has made superbugs a global issue, with their proliferation increasing every day at an alarming rate.

The hidden pandemic of superbugs could end medicine. This is the simple truth. If you think I'm exaggerating, let's consider the facts.

Antibiotics are crucial for protecting the health of individuals both in India and worldwide. The first person to receive the first antibiotic, penicillin, had developed an infection after scratching the side of his face while pruning roses: he died when his supply of the miracle drug ran out. We might be going back to a period where even minor scratches pose lethal risks. Additionally, diseases like tuberculosis (TB), pneumonia, gonorrhoea, and even seemingly minor infections like strep throat may become untreatable.

People with chronic conditions like diabetes, which affects over 100 million people in India alone, are susceptible to infections due to weakened immune systems. Further, cancer patients receiving chemotherapy are at a high risk of developing serious infections. Recipients of organ transplant and those undergoing dialysis for advanced kidney disease also face a heightened risk of infection. Thus, antibiotics play a vital role in protecting these vulnerable populations – and modern medicine requires antibiotics that work.

Preface

Sepsis, a response to infections typically caused by bacteria, affects at least 11 million Indians every year and often results in death. It's especially prevalent in ICUs in India, where up to half of the patients may develop it. Patients undergoing surgery risk life-threatening infections, and antibiotics are necessary for surgical procedures to be viable. This is particularly important for the growing number of Caesarean sections, which account for about one in every five births in India.

India is at the forefront of the global battle against superbugs. In India, in 2019, superbugs were directly responsible for around 300,000 deaths and were a contributing factor to one million more. The confluence of India's dense population, environmental challenges, inadequate sanitation, and healthcare systems, as well as low levels of public awareness of this problem, creates a fertile ground for the spread of superbugs. The situation is exacerbated by the easy over-the-counter availability of antibiotics, leading to widespread self-medication and a general tendency among healthcare providers to prescribe antibiotics as a go-to solution. Additionally, the market is flooded with untested and unapproved combinations of antibiotics.

India's role as a major producer of pharmaceuticals, including antibiotics, adds another layer of complexity to the problem. Cities like Hyderabad, known for their pharmaceutical industries, have reported dangerously high concentrations of antibiotics in local waterbodies. This

Preface

problem extends to many of India's urban and industrial areas, such as Delhi, where antibiotics are found in both water supply and sewage systems.

Surprisingly, around 70 per cent of medically important antibiotics sold in the world are not used in human health but to plump up animals for consumption. In 2020, India ranked among the top five countries, along with China, Brazil, the US, and Australia, in terms of antibiotic usage for livestock including cattle, sheep, chickens, and pigs.

Tackling the superbug crisis requires a multifaceted approach that goes beyond the reach of only doctors and scientists. While these experts play a critical role in advising on policy and revising prescription practices, a broader societal effort is needed to combat the spread of superbugs. In response to this growing threat, in 2022, India, along with thirty-eight other countries, committed to a significant reduction in the use of antibiotics in animal agriculture by 30 per cent to 50 per cent by the end of the decade.

To address the root causes of antibiotic resistance, it's essential to enforce stricter regulations on pharmaceutical companies to prevent dumping antibiotic waste into the environment. Physicians must resist the urge to prescribe antibiotics without a diagnosis of a treatable bacterial infection. Similarly, pharmacies must be regulated to limit the sale of antibiotics to only those with prescriptions. Crucially, public awareness and behaviour, must also change. Educating the public about the risks of antibiotic misuse and the importance of not demanding antibiotics for minor illnesses is vital.

This challenge is for all of us. In this book, I will inform readers about the remarkable discovery of antibiotics, the consequences of their misuse that led to the terrifying emergence of superbugs, and the actions we can collectively take to safeguard the future of modern medicine and our own well-being.

Perhaps one way to understand the dimension of the danger is by comparison to the most recent global pandemic. The mayhem caused by COVID-19 is well known. We all bear the trauma of the pandemic years. Many of us will need time to heal. Others will try to forget about it as soon as possible.

Many of us are also acquainted with some of the major challenges facing humanity such as climate change, the threat of a close encounter with an asteroid, and rogue artificial intelligence. But another insidious threat hides in plain sight in our daily lives and that is the silent, or hidden, pandemic of superbugs. We ignore this calamity at our peril.

A hundred years ago, infectious diseases were one of the leading causes of death worldwide. The use of antibiotics and the implementation of modern public health measures, such as vaccinations, sanitation, and improved living conditions, have since significantly reduced the impact of infectious diseases on global mortality. Today, this trend is being reversed.

The writing is on the wall. Today, superbugs present a

greater threat than COVID-19. If left unchecked, they will inflict a heavier burden on the economy and result in a more significant loss of life. It is clear to me that the discussion of antibiotic-resistant superbugs needs to move beyond microbiology conferences and conversations with doctors in white coats. It needs to move from the corridors of hospitals into the chat groups of ordinary citizens and into the halls of power.

To understand the superbug pandemic, we must examine our relationship with antibiotics because the two are deeply interconnected. The discovery and subsequent widespread use of antibiotics revolutionized modern medicine. The golden age of discovery of antibiotics lasted from the discovery of penicillin in 1928 to around 1964. The rate of discovery and development of antibiotics slowed over the next sixty years. The slowdown is often referred to as the 'innovation gap' in antibiotic research, and today, there are not nearly enough antibiotics for deadly superbugs.

Overreliance on and misuse of these drugs have given rise to superbugs. Today we are faced with a crisis, since many of these wonder drugs don't work any more. **The last new major class of antibiotics that reached the market was daptomycin, discovered in 1984 and approved for use nearly two decades later.**

No truly innovative antibiotics have hit the market in over twenty years. At the same time, bacteria that are resistant to every one of the antibiotics we have at our disposal are

When the Drugs Don't Work

Year of introduction of common antibiotics and year when credible reports of antibiotic resistance were first reported

Antibiotic	Antibiotic Deployed to the Public	Antibiotic Resistance
Penicillin G	1942	1947
Streptomycin	1944	1946
Chloramphenicol	1948	1950
Erythromycin	1952	1955
Tetracycline	1952	1959
Vancomycin	1956	1982
Cephalosporins	1964	1982
Linezolid	2000	2001
Daptomycin	2003	2006
Ceftolozane/Tazobactam	2014	2021

Table modified from data from the United Nations Environment Programme report *Bracing for superbugs: Strengthening environmental action in the One Health response to antimicrobial resistance* (2023).

Other sources may provide somewhat different dates based on the country of deployment of the antibiotic and the criteria for determining resistance.

showing up with alarming frequency. Superbugs resistant to multiple antibiotics are moving from being increasingly difficult to tackle to being impossible to treat. The words of an infectious diseases specialist breaking the news to a patient who had acquired a superbug infection after an amputation still ring in my ears: 'We don't know how to treat you.'

Antibiotics are used in almost every sphere of our lives. If they stop working, it will truly be the end of modern medicine. Let me tell you about two personal events that occurred during the writing of this book which illustrate my own complex relationship with antibiotics.

My eleven-year-old son came home from school one day feeling sick. He developed a fever the next day and a sore throat with a cough. These respiratory symptoms are common, but they're also non-specific and tell us nothing about the cause of illness. We tested for COVID-19 at home with a rapid antigen kit, which came back negative. Appreciating that most respiratory infections that kids pick up get better on their own, my son rested at home for the next few days and drank plenty of fluids. The only medicine we gave him was a low dose of a fever reducer available without a prescription

When the symptoms had not resolved in a week, we took him to his paediatrician, who tested for COVID-19 again, influenza A and B, and the bacterium that causes strep throat. These tests are usually accurate if they render a positive result but are less reliable when the results come back negative. My son tested negative in all cases.

And so, we were no closer to identifying the cause of my son's ailment. And it wasn't getting better. What's worth noting is that the paediatrician did not prescribe any medicine, but instead asked us to keep monitoring symptoms and come back if they worsened or didn't get better on their own. What the paediatrician *did not do* was prescribe an antibiotic.

My son could have been suffering from an infection that was not routinely tested for, or from allergies, or another ailment for which there were no rapid tests. More accurate cultures could have confirmed if there was indeed a bacterial infection. But thankfully for us, and as you might have expected, my son did get better on his own.

My spouse and I are well aware of the dangers of over-prescription of antibiotics. We currently live in the US where antibiotics are not available without prescriptions. A similar situation with a different child, parent, or physician might have played out differently in a different time or in a different part of the world. We could have pushed the physician to prescribe an antibiotic. Additionally, she might also have been expected to prescribe an antibiotic or two, even if the chance that they were needed was low.

Rapid diagnostic tests might not have been available or been more expensive than antibiotics. Also, they are not entirely accurate. When the gold standard for identifying bacteria and matching them to antibiotics that work against them takes two days or more, a physician must move beyond the textbook to apply practical experience. They must consider the resources they have at their disposal, what other infections they have seen recently, and whether the patient is likely to wait for a confirmatory diagnosis. A physician might ask themselves the question: 'Will I ever see this patient again?'

When antibiotics first went into broad use starting in the 1950s, it was common for physicians to prescribe antibiotics not after the confirmation of a bacterial cause, but simply by observing symptoms. Even then, it was appreciated that most respiratory infections are not caused by bacteria. As such, antibiotics that have specificity against bacteria are useless in treating infections caused by viruses or seasonal allergies. In fact, as we will see, they can be harmful not only to broader society, but also to the person who takes them.

More recently, around 60–80 per cent of patients treated for COVID-19 were prescribed an antibiotic, such as a cephalosporin or azithromycin. This was despite the common knowledge that these antibiotics are not effective against the coronavirus that causes COVID-19. Even if physicians suspected that there was an associated bacterial infection lurking alongside the coronavirus, they would've known that the odds of such a co-infection were small. According to a recent study, only 5 per cent of patients had both the coronavirus and a bacterial infection treatable with an antibiotic.

What about the parents of a sick child? In countries like India where many antibiotics are easily available without a prescription, parents watching a suffering child may be tempted to get them from a local pharmacy themselves and give them without an understanding of whether they are required or how they work. They may remember a time when they popped antibiotics for a couple of days and got better and assumed that it was the antibiotics that had healed them. We tend to overestimate the effect of actions we take. As a result, action, even if taken without a logical basis, despite being actively harmful, is often seen as preferable to inaction. I understand the urge.

The second incident I want to highlight occurred recently, when I was having a conversation with my aunt. A resilient woman well into her seventies, she had weathered a litany of health challenges over the years. As the conversation flowed, the topic of this book surfaced. My aunt shared an unsettling belief that she had become resistant to antibiotics. She felt there was an inherent flaw within her, making her vulnerable to infections that antibiotics could not remedy.

This misconception struck a chord with me. It was not the first time I had encountered the sentiment, and it made me realize why this book needed to be written. I explained to my aunt that our bodies do not become resistant to antibiotics. Instead, antibiotics are ineffective in treating infections caused by the resistant bacteria that are inside us.

I also explained to my aunt that not all bacteria are harmful: there are trillions of bacteria inside us that contribute positively to our health. These beneficial bacteria inhabit various parts of our bodies like the gut, skin, and mouth. They assist in digesting food, producing essential vitamins, regulating our immune responses, and even influencing our mood and mental health. Beyond these beneficial bacteria, a significant number remain neutral, causing neither harm nor providing any explicit benefit.

This nuanced relationship with bacteria stands in contrast to our interactions with viruses. Let's consider COVID-19, a viral disease. There's never a circumstance in which the presence of the causative coronavirus in a human body is considered normal or natural. Whether it manifests with pronounced symptoms or remains silent, it is an invasion by a foreign entity. The virus exists to replicate and spread at the host's expense.

Many harmless bacteria can become disease-causing given the opportunity. Some may enter from outside, but many others live within our bodies. When disease-causing bacteria acquire resistance to antibiotics, they become superbugs.

Here's the sobering reality: we will never completely eliminate superbugs because bacteria living within us can develop antibiotic resistance. But there's a silver lining. By reshaping our approach to antibiotics and understanding our relationship with bacteria, we can change the narrative. The pandemic of superbugs looms large, but the future isn't set in stone.

Through this book, we will consider the causes – that's plural – of the superbug crisis. Make no mistake, there is no single cause or simple solution. One of the many reasons is the overprescription of antibiotics, a significant driver of the rise of superbugs. Unnecessary exposure to antibiotics gives bacteria a chance to adapt and become resistant. Agriculture exacerbates the issue, with the overuse of antibiotics in livestock and fish farming. These antibiotics then enter the environment and the food chain, leading to widespread exposure and again, the evolution of superbugs.

Poor infection control leads to the rapid spread of superbugs. This is worsened by substandard hygiene and sanitation practices in communities. Here, communities and governments also play a vital role in stopping the spread of superbugs. Policymakers must enforce stricter regulations to curtail the rampant overuse of antibiotics and also to incentivize the development of new drugs. The pharmaceutical industry needs to prioritize and accelerate research on superbugs and the next generation of antibiotics.

Ultimately, as individuals we must embed good habits in our daily life, such as refraining from self-prescribing antibiotics or veering from a recommended prescription course. Just as we teach our children to look both ways before they cross the street and drill it into them until the habit becomes instinct, we need to drill it into everyone that antibiotics must be used with caution until that idea becomes instinct. This is essential to combat superbugs and slow down the rise of antibiotic resistance.

1

A Daily Tragedy

'Every medicine, every antibiotic they gave her, it did nothing. Her body was tiny, but her battle was immense.' Anjali struggled to maintain her composure as she retold her daughter's story for the documentary film's crew. 'As a mother, you feel so helpless.'

Anjali's daughter was born prematurely and spent a heart-wrenching seven days in the ICU of a hospital in Amravati, a small town in Maharashtra. Those seven days were filled with a roller coaster of emotions for Anjali: hope, despair, and a mother's fervent prayers. Yet, despite the valiant efforts of the medical team, a parent's worst nightmare came true for her and her family. The tiny girl died, before she could even leave the hospital, before she had been introduced to the world. She had not even been named.

The paediatrician who treated Anjali's newborn was reflective, but gave a telling assessment of the tragedy. The baby died of neonatal sepsis, a life-threatening medical condition which occurs when a newborn acquires a severe infection that spreads throughout the body. The infection was caused by an untreatable bacterial strain – a superbug that didn't respond to any antibiotic. There was nothing that could've been done to save the baby.

Sadly, this tragedy is far from an isolated incident in India today. Anjali's daughter is one of the approximately 60,000 babies in the country who die each year from infections caused by bacteria that don't respond to front-line antibiotics. These superbugs threaten to upend modern medicine and push back decades of progress in improving the quality of life in India.

'What happened to me shouldn't happen to anyone else. It's a pain you can't put into words,' says Anjali, her voice tinged with a sorrow that she knows will never completely go away.

Unfortunately, we are heading towards a catastrophe in which many mothers like Anjali will regularly mourn the loss of their children. India is at the forefront of a crisis, a hidden pandemic of superbugs, that is killing our most vulnerable populations. We must act now or face the consequences because we have created this crisis. Unfortunately, there is a lack of public awareness about how we got here and what we can do to solve the problem.

A Daily Tragedy

This book covers the tragic circumstances of the decisions that brought us to this point, the dangers we face, and what we need to do to emerge from this dark shadow that threatens to take healthcare back into the pre-antibiotic era.

However, before we talk about superbugs, we need to acknowledge how much life has improved in the last few decades for most of us. India, now the most populous country in the world, has witnessed a healthcare transformation that is nothing short of miraculous. Consider this: if you were born in India around Independence, you could expect to live only until your early thirties. Life was fraught with challenges such as malnutrition, inadequate sanitation, and widespread infectious diseases.

Fast forward to the present, and the average Indian can expect to live up to around the age of seventy, a monumental advance. And while today there are indeed large disparities between genders, communities, and economic classes, the overall progress we have made in improving the lives of common people is undeniable. We must take a step back and appreciate this.

There isn't one single benign factor that led to this revolution, but rather many things working in tandem. Better education and economic progress played an important role in health awareness. An educated populace can make more informed choices. Economic progress has also enabled advances in health. Further, knowledge without the capability to act is futile, and that ability came from relative advances in prosperity, which allowed for improved well-being in successive generations.

Then there's what we eat. Enhanced diets significantly reduced malnutrition and starvation, leading to healthier and longer lives. India has not experienced a single serious famine since its independence. The Green Revolution of the 1960s and 1970s helped the country significantly increase its agricultural production through the introduction of high-yielding crop varieties and modern farming techniques. This allowed India to not only feed itself, but to post annual surpluses for many staple crops, and even become a food exporter.

It's not easy to transform the infrastructure of a country, but India has persevered on this front too. Improvements in sanitation and sewage systems have made living conditions cleaner, reducing the risk of diseases. While open defecation remains a persistent issue, strides have been made to reduce it.

Let's not forget healthcare. From basic medical centres to specialized hospitals, the quality of medical facilities and professionals has seen a marked improvement in the country. More can and should be done, but we should appreciate the efforts of healthcare professionals in modern India. Take cholera, for example. Historically, six of the seven cholera pandemics that occurred globally originated in India before Independence. However, not a single cholera pandemic has occurred in India in the past few decades. While smaller cholera outbreaks do still occur, the risk of contracting cholera and dying from it has greatly diminished.

These facts are not just academic for me. My family, like millions of others, benefited from this progress. We were lifted out of poverty and joined many others as part of the 'Great Indian Story'. My father was born before Independence in a village that had no electricity. He grew up without access to clean water and sanitary sewage disposal. Despite meagre means, he went on to complete his education at one of India's premier medical institutions, the All India Institute of Medical Sciences, which was founded in New Delhi in 1956. My mother also came from a similar background. She received her postgraduate medical degree from the same institution. Their education prepared them for further training abroad, after which they returned to treat patients at a district town in India.

Although my own story took a slightly different path, there are some similarities. Like my parents before me, my own education was almost entirely subsidized by the Indian taxpayer. Although the following statement might sound fantastic, I've crunched the numbers, and it is absolutely true: the total cost of my college education to my family was less than that of a high-end smartphone today. This number neglects to account for inflation of course, but it is still a startling realization.

When I arrived in the US to continue my studies in microbiology, the move was made possible by the generous fellowships I received, and the research grants awarded to my mentor and PhD adviser. I did not have to pay for doctoral training. Indeed, this is why I have always felt indebted to taxpayers in two countries.

The benefits of widespread vaccination are also personal for me. My father nearly died from a severe smallpox infection while he was in college. I was born the same year that *Roti, Kapada, Aur Makaan* (translated to Food, Clothes, and Shelter in Hindi) with Manoj Kumar in a lead role and the up-and-coming Amitabh Bachchan in a supporting role was the biggest Hindi blockbuster. Later, I would be immunized around the same time that the last known case of smallpox was reported in the country in 1975. Born after smallpox was eradicated, my son has never needed to be vaccinated against it. Polio is no longer the concern it once was in India either.

Even for other diseases that have not been eradicated, vaccination drives have substantially reduced mortality. Fresh in public memory is the massive COVID-19 vaccination drive that India launched to ensure citizens were protected. Today, India not only vaccinates its own but produces many of the vaccines used around the world.

If vaccines have helped prevent some infectious diseases, then antibiotics have treated other persistent ones. Ask anyone what some of the greatest advances of the past century are and you might hear answers that include the personal computer and internet revolution, global air travel, and television. But let me offer a serious contender. Antibiotics are among the greatest technological triumphs in human history. Without question, these drugs are an indispensable aspect of modern life, transforming once-fatal bacterial infections into manageable conditions.

Do you think I'm exaggerating? Antibiotics are the drugs that made modern medicine possible. Before antibiotics existed, a scratch or a scraped knee could result in a deadly infection. Today, antibiotics are used preventatively in surgeries, to treat chronic conditions like cystic fibrosis, and to stave off infections in high-risk scenarios. They have saved uncounted millions of lives, and an estimated 40 billion doses of these medicines are consumed every year.

But the pressing and unavoidable question remains: what do we do if and when these life-saving drugs become ineffective?

When bacteria develop resistance to antibiotics, everyday medical procedures become high-risk. Childbirth and the initial months of a baby's life turn precarious. Even routine hospital visits and minor surgeries carry significant danger. Simply housing patients together in the same ward introduces risk.

If bacteria that are resistant to many, or all the available, antibiotics spread widely, it isn't just a minor or temporary setback, it is a public health crisis. The rise of antibiotic-resistant superbugs adversely affects life expectancy. The consequences are severe, putting immense pressure on healthcare systems and in India, it rolls back the clock on the hard-won medical advances of the past few decades.

But it is time to brace yourself. This dystopian future is not a hypothetical scenario: it's already manifesting right now. In recent years, a worrying trend has emerged – there are an increasing number of powerful superbug variants of bacteria that were treatable with antibiotics just a few years ago but have now grown resistant to them.

From around 1950, there was always a backup antibiotic that physicians could resort to. When bacteria gained resistance to one class of antibiotics, physicians moved on to the next one. But there is now an ongoing race, one that humanity is losing. In recent years, superbugs have been gaining the upper hand, and the medicine cabinet is running bare. As a result, patients are dying of untreatable infections. And what's worse is the pipeline is also running dry. No new major class of antibiotics has been made commercially available in decades, and we are close to entering the post-antibiotic era.

You might ask how this is possible. In nearly every other realm of science and technology, as time passes and we learn more, we get better at doing things. Moore's Law (which states that the processing power of a computer doubles every few years) is a famous observation that explains why the smartphone in my pocket is much more powerful than the guidance computer used to land the first humans on the moon in 1969.

Natural Selection of Antibiotic-Resistant Bacteria

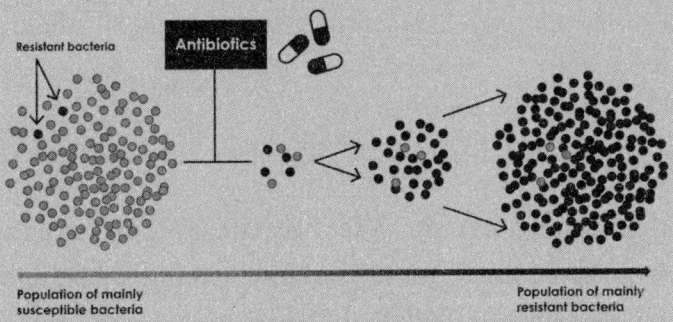

Image credit: The ReAct toolbox on 'mutations and selection'

Initial Population: Initially, there is a diverse population of bacteria, most of which are susceptible to antibiotics (represented by the grey dots). A few bacteria are naturally resistant due to random mutations that exist in populations (shown here in black).

Application of Antibiotics: When antibiotics are introduced (the pills icon), they kill most of the susceptible bacteria. Resistant bacteria survive because they have certain traits that protect them from the effects of the drug.

Multiplication of Resistant Bacteria: The resistant bacteria (black dots) survive the antibiotic treatment. Since the susceptible ones (grey dots) are now largely eliminated, the resistant bacteria face less competition for resources and can multiply freely.

> **Change in Population**: Over time, as resistant bacteria replicate, the population shifts from being mostly susceptible to being primarily composed of resistant bacteria. This means the antibiotic is now much less effective since most of the bacteria present can tolerate it.

But nature has a secret advantage over machines. Carbon-based life forms have extra capabilities that silicon-based transistors don't have: they can evolve. Life has had plenty of time to figure out how to do things better than humans.

Even when we find ways to defeat bacteria, they come back. A new generation of bacteria can grow very fast – some even double in population every twenty minutes. Bacteria are incredibly versatile, and they've been here for billions of years. Modern microbiology is not even a few hundred years old, and does not have much of a chance against these formidable foes. British chemist Lesley Orgel aptly summed up this dynamic with his observation: 'Evolution is cleverer than you are.'

Now, I will let you in on another little secret. Humans can make great smartphones and rocket ships, but so far, our track record at making drugs that beat bacteria is pretty lousy. Technically, antibiotics are natural products made by the bacteria and moulds that can kill or retard the growth of certain bacteria. Sometimes, the definitions are broadened to

A Daily Tragedy

include natural products that kill fungi or parasites, but we'll stick to the original definition for clarity.

What about drugs that chemists design and make from scratch? To differentiate them from antibiotics, we will call these synthetic compounds antibacterials. There are not as many antibacterials as there are antibiotics. In fact, most of the antibiotics in use even today are ones we took from (mostly soil) bacteria. We've tinkered with antibiotics that soil bacteria naturally make to produce them at scale, improve their effectiveness, and make them last a little bit longer. But massive projects to create antibacterials from scratch have little to show for the money and effort that have been put into them. That's one of the reasons that most major pharmaceutical companies have moved on from the effort to create new antibacterials altogether. Nature is still the best weapon against nature.

I can trace the first shoots of my inspiration for writing this book back to 2010. In August of that year, a scientific article in the medical journal *The Lancet Infectious Diseases* became the unlikely subject of discussion across India, even making its way to Parliament. The research article described the spread of a gene and an enzyme that gave bacterial resistance to certain antibiotics, making them superbugs. It was named NDM-1 after New Delhi. Perhaps you vaguely remember the controversy even if you've forgotten the details.

During the next few months, the issue (or non-issue depending on who you asked) of antibiotic resistance and superbugs gained significant attention from high-profile medical experts on traditional and social media in India and elsewhere. Soon, politicians got into the act as well. Much was written at the time, but it was impossible to know what would follow. We did not know how NDM-1 would spread or how serious it would become.

Fourteen years have passed since that initial episode with NDM-1, and it is natural to wonder what has happened. Were the *Lancet Infectious Diseases* authors making a huge fuss over something that wasn't a real threat? The truth is that good science takes time. Experiments are conducted and results are formulated methodically. Ideas are discussed and debated, often over a span of years. New studies refine, dispel, or build on previous work. Science has no chance to compete when pitted against the news cycle which strives to find the latest controversy to attract eyeballs and online engagement. The topic was buried and forgotten.

No doubt media outlets do sometimes mention antibiotic resistance when there's a specific incident. But there's rarely the time or space to delve into any details or to provide context. You would think that every incident is isolated, but it's not.

The second spark for writing this book came in 2016 with the publication of an influential report that you've probably never heard of. The report titled 'Tackling Drug-resistant Infections Globally' by the Review on Antimicrobial Resistance framed the problem of superbugs and their terrible impact on health and economy in stark terms. This study was commissioned by the government of the UK, and it was informally dubbed the O'Neill Report after the economist Jim O'Neill who chaired the Review.

In 2014, the then prime minister of the UK, David Cameron, asked O'Neill to survey the scale of the problem of resistance, which isn't simply a health crisis, but potentially a long-term economic calamity that could derail global development and security. O'Neill was no stranger to discerning current trends and tying them together to create a big picture. While at the investment bank Goldman Sachs, he had coined the acronym BRIC to refer to Brazil, Russia, India, and China after identifying them as emerging powerhouses poised for economic growth. As chair of the Review on Antimicrobial Resistance, he immediately commissioned expert teams at consultancy firms to come to terms with the economic underpinnings of this worldwide menace.

Before moving on, I need to clarify a few terms. Antimicrobials are a group of substances including antibiotics, antivirals, antifungals, and antiseptics. These are powerful tools in the arsenal of modern medicine. Antibiotics are a subset of natural antimicrobials that work on specific bacteria.

Let's be very clear. As a class of drugs, antibiotics work against bacteria. They are ineffective against viruses. In addition, some antibiotics are geared to act against specific bacteria and not all of them. To treat a viral infection, we'd need to be prescribed a very specific antiviral. And to treat fungi, we'd need to be prescribed an antifungal. Each class of drug works only because of the very distinct biology of its target.

Bacterial resistance is part of a broader scheme of antimicrobial resistance. Apart from bacteria, many other microbes (such as disease-causing fungi) develop defences against the effects of antimicrobials. In this book, we narrow our focus to the bacterial superbugs which present the main threats to conventional antibiotics. Fungi are also spreading and developing resistance, but that is perhaps the subject of another book.

The O'Neill report found that if left unchecked, by 2050, the problem of antimicrobial resistance could inflict a staggering cost of US$100 trillion on the global economy – an economic apocalypse by any measure. For comparison, this would correspond to a loss equivalent to roughly nearly 4 per cent of the annual global gross domestic product by 2050. It would cast an estimated 28 million people into poverty and swell annual healthcare costs.

The report also predicted that by 2050, 10 million people would die from antimicrobial resistance every year. Of this number, 7.5 million would die from bacterial infections caused by superbugs. To put that large number in perspective, that is more people than currently die from cancer. Even this number probably didn't account for the true toll from secondary impacts like compromised surgeries and increased vulnerability to epidemics.

Let me put it another way. The World Health Organization (WHO) estimates that around 15 million people in all died directly or indirectly from COVID-19 across 2020 and 2021, the two deadliest years of the coronavirus pandemic. So, on the current trajectory, antimicrobial resistance is poised to be more devastating and more unrelentingly lethal than the most lethal pandemic of our lifetimes. In fact, the WHO reports that antimicrobial resistance is among the top global public health threats facing humanity.

O'Neill made several urgent recommendations.

First, a global public awareness campaign needed to educate the populace, particularly the younger generation, about the dangers of antibiotic resistance.

Second, financial incentives needed to be set in place to drive the creation of new antibiotics. Estimating the cost of bringing a new antibiotic to market, the report proposed that market entry rewards of around US$1 billion for each new antibiotic would be suitable.

Third, technological advances needed to be made in rapid diagnosis so that drugs could be pinpointed to target specific bacteria.

In agriculture, where antibiotics are frequently overused, better surveillance and national targets were recommended to guide more responsible usage. Restricting or banning use of antibiotics crucial for human health in animals was another recommendation. The review called on wealthy countries to do their fair share and to take the lead, recommending that all antibiotic prescriptions be guided by rapid diagnostic tests and up-to-date surveillance.

The O'Neill report which outlined the shape of the impending crisis with antimicrobial resistance was discussed among policymakers and politicians. It provided quotable statistics for microbiologists like me. But much like other position papers and policy reports, it failed to capture the imagination of the broader public including taxpayers and the politicians who determine how to allocate tax revenues.

If the O'Neill report was a wake-up-call that few heeded, then a study published in 2022 in *The Lancet*, one of the world's most prestigious medical journals, by a global consortium of antimicrobial resistance collaborators should've been a slap in the face. This study in *The Lancet* study didn't extrapolate bacterial resistance into the future – it convincingly showed that this is already a very real and present danger. It synthesized data from 204 countries and territories and painted an unsettling picture. For the first time, we had reliable estimates of the death toll from superbugs. Not only were the numbers bad, but they were a lot worse than expected.

In 2019 alone, nearly 1.3 million people died directly from antibiotic-resistant infections. In total, antibiotic resistance contributed to almost 5 million deaths that year from complications. What this indicated was that we were two-thirds of the way to the estimated 7.5 million annual deaths from bacterial infections by 2050 in the O'Neill report. So, if anything, the O'Neill assumptions might well have been an underestimate.

What *The Lancet* study had also found was that antibiotic-resistant bacteria already cause more deaths than HIV/AIDS, TB, or malaria. The toll is especially high among the youngest: one in five of these deaths occurred in children under the age of five. The study also provided a clear indication of the worst culprits. Six bacteria that can thwart antibiotics used to treat illnesses were estimated to have caused 80 per cent of the fatal infections from antimicrobial resistance. These superbugs are *Escherichia coli* (often just called *E. coli*), *Staphylococcus aureus, Klebsiella pneumoniae, Streptococcus pneumoniae, Acinetobacter baumannii,* and *Pseudomonas aeruginosa.*

Together, these six pathogens were linked to over 3.5 million deaths in 2019. I will refer to them as the 'Deadly Six' superbugs, and they will show up repeatedly in this book. Out of these six, one superbug, methicillin-resistant *Staphylococcus aureus* has its own nickname, 'Mersa' after the abbreviation MRSA.

Despite these alarming facts and figures, the public remains largely oblivious to the scale and urgency of the problem of antibiotic-resistant superbugs. You may even be asking yourself this: if the threat of superbugs is so severe, why don't we hear more about it? It's an important question that strikes at the heart of why the rise of superbugs is a hidden danger and a silent pandemic. I don't think there's a single good reason for this low-key response. Here's what I do know though. When I wrote *COVID-19: Separating Fact from Fiction*, I had to explain the trajectory of a pandemic for a virus with a relatively simple biology. The fact of the matter is, the problem of superbugs is far more complex and more difficult to get across, in terms of lay understanding, and of course, it is far more difficult to research and counteract as well.

Bacteria are cellular organisms with far more complex life cycles than viruses. A single kind of coronavirus caused the COVID-19 pandemic. In contrast, there's not one disease-causing superbug we can point to as the sole cause of deaths due to antibiotic resistance.

I mentioned the Deadly Six superbugs we will focus on in this book. But there are many other bacteria such as multidrug-resistant (MDR) TB that are also lethal. I've chosen to focus on a subset here, but the problem is there isn't a single culprit: there's a whole host of characters that are potential superbugs.

While the coronavirus that caused the COVID-19 pandemic was a virus we had never seen before, the bacteria that develop resistance and turn into superbugs live among us. This adds an additional level of complexity in explaining and understanding the threat.

2

Superbug Signatures

Imagine a bustling city where everyone goes about their daily lives in harmony. Suddenly, one day, an outsider enters this city and creates chaos. If you think about it, this is somewhat like what happened with the novel coronavirus that caused the COVID-19 pandemic.

However, it's an entirely different challenge when some residents of that city, who've lived there peacefully for years suddenly change their behaviour and become threats. This is the situation with bacteria like *E. coli*, which can turn into a harmful superbug after living harmlessly in our bodies for years.

Not all bacteria that belong to the same species are superbugs either. In other words, not all disease-causing *E. coli* are superbugs. It's the resistance genes that power up a disease-causing strain of *E. coli* in a person that makes it an

E. coli superbug. Let's call these supergenes because that's essentially what they are.

In the standard superhero story, an ordinary person is bestowed with superhuman powers after some kind of mishap. I think it helps to imagine superbugs as the microbial equivalent. Antibiotic resistance is essentially the story of ordinary bacteria picking up supergenes that turn them into superbugs. And the more supergenes they acquire, the more sinister they become as fewer antibiotics work against them. It is crucial to understand this to make sense of the problem of antibiotic resistance.

We met the Deadly Six superbugs in the previous chapter. It is time to tell you that four of the six are known as 'Gram-negative' bacteria. As we will discuss, these are particularly difficult to beat because they have figured out multiple different ways to thwart the antibiotics we throw at them.

What's worth noting about superbugs is that it's not the bacteria themselves that are untreatable; it's their acquisition of multiple supergenes. These confer the resistance that transforms them into invulnerable killers.

Broadly, resistant bacteria fall into three different categories of superbugs that sound like they came out of a horrible branding exercise for various models of a car. Bacteria can be tested for their susceptibility. Superbugs are bacteria that are not susceptible to at least a few antibiotics – in other words, they are resistant to these.

MDR bacteria are superbugs that can combat at least one

antibiotic in three or more categories, rendering multiple treatments ineffective. Next up are extensively drug-resistant (XDR) bacteria which are superbugs whose defences have been honed to the point where they are resistant to all but two antibiotic categories. Most frightening are pandrug-resistant (PDR) bacteria, which are medical nightmares since these are resistant to nearly all or all commercially available antibiotics. The Deadly Six have elite superbug status because they can pick up many genes that make them resistant to many antibiotics, and they can cause life-threatening infections.

There's more. Bacteria can grow really fast. They pass on their traits to their offspring in the familiar parent-to-child way like mammals and reptiles. This is how natural antibiotic resistance that arises spontaneously can spread.

But here's the wild part that is entirely different from us: bacteria can also directly share special traits with each other through mobile genetic elements, even if they aren't parent and child. This is often how they spread those powerful traits that make some of them superbugs. This process is known as horizontal gene transfer. Mobile elements and horizontal gene transfer play crucial roles in the development of antibiotic resistance and the emergence of superbugs.

Bacteria have a single circular chromosome. In addition to the chromosome, they often contain plasmids, which are smaller loops of DNA. These plasmids are significant because they can be easily acquired from other bacteria or the environment, and they can carry genes that provide resistance to antibiotics. Plasmids replicate independently of the bacterial chromosome, and a single bacterial cell can contain numerous copies of a plasmid.

Plasmids also often carry antibiotic resistance genes, which weren't common in plasmids before the widespread use of antibiotics. Today, plasmids carrying genes that offer protection against various antibiotics have become more prevalent. Often a single plasmid carries multiple antibiotic resistance genes. In such cases, the presence of one antibiotic can help a superbug maintain resistance to several antibiotics since all of the genes are carried on the same plasmid.

A daydreaming microbiologist can imagine how this ability might be beneficial to humans. Say, for example, you're on a bus, and the person sitting next to you has a unique ability – she never catches a cold. What if, just by sitting next to her, you could suddenly gain that same ability? Or imagine that you're in a classroom sitting next to someone exceptionally good at mathematics. Now, rather than studying for years, what if you could just tap them on the shoulder and instantly gain their ability?

While these analogies help paint a picture, they aren't perfect comparisons. In our examples, there isn't a pressing need for you to avoid catching a cold, or to master mathematics overnight. But for bacteria, having antibiotic resistance supergenes can be crucial, especially when someone is taking antibiotics. It might be the difference between the bacteria

Superbug Signatures

How Bacteria Share Their Superpowers

Mobile Genetic Elements

Plasmids
Circles of DNA that can move between cells.

Transposons
Small pieces of DNA that can go into and change the overall DNA of a cell. These can move from chromosomes (which carry all the genes essential for germ survival) to plasmids and back.

Phages
Viruses that attack germs and can carry DNA from germ to germ.

How Mobile Genetic Elements Work

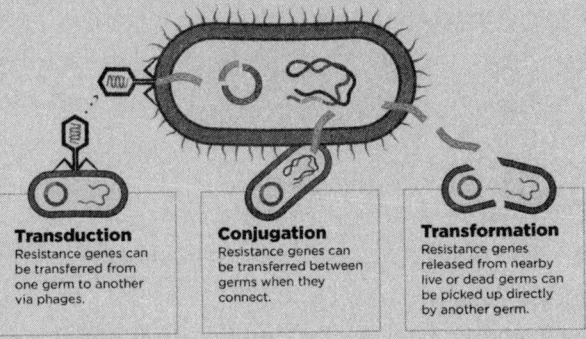

Transduction
Resistance genes can be transferred from one germ to another via phages.

Conjugation
Resistance genes can be transferred between germs when they connect.

Transformation
Resistance genes released from nearby live or dead germs can be picked up directly by another germ.

Image credit: CDC

Tiny Loops with Big Impact: Plasmids are tiny loops of DNA inside bacterial cells that can be packed with information, including on fending off antibiotics. What makes them extraordinary is their ability to move from one bacterium to another.

Jumping Genes: Transposons are bits of DNA that can jump from one place to another within a bacterium's genetic material. Sometimes, they land within a plasmid, hitching a ride to a new bacterium.

> **The Viral Couriers:** Bacteriophages, or phages for short, are viruses that infect bacteria. They can accidentally package bacterial DNA, including resistance genes, into their viral particles. When they infect the next bacterium, they deliver these genes.
>
> Mobile genetic elements supercharge resistance spread. In **transduction**, phages pick up and deliver resistance genes from one bacterium to another. In **conjugation**, bacteria form a physical bridge to exchange plasmids loaded with resistance genes. In **transformation**, bacteria grab bits of DNA left in the environment by living and dead bacteria including antibiotic resistance genes.

surviving or dying. Essentially, the stakes are much higher for the bacteria than in our analogies.

Horizontal gene transfer is a key reason we have to worry about bacteria sharing supergenes. They can just 'tap' into other bacteria and acquire resistance traits, making them even more challenging to combat. Resistance genes that arise in one part of the world can spread in shared environments and make it to different parts of the world.

As if things weren't bad enough, these supergenes aren't just shared by the same kind of bacteria, they are also shared across different species. All of a sudden, the *E. coli* which was harmless in the gut can cause disease and also pick up a mobile snippet of DNA containing a supergene that makes it invincible against antibiotics. This *E. coli* superbug strain then passes this supergene baton to another disease-causing bacterium like *Klebsiella* which is in the neighbourhood. Suddenly, you have two different bacteria that have developed resistance, fanning the flames of superbug spread.

There's yet another reason that the problem of superbugs is underappreciated. Even though nearly 80 per cent of deaths they cause occur due to infections initially in the abdomen, chest, and bloodstream, superbug attacks aren't confined to a single part of the body. Not having a single site of infection makes it harder to explain or understand the threat or to mount a concerted response. The *E. coli* that was living harmoniously in your gut can make it to your urinary tract to cause a terrible infection. The *Pseudomonas aeruginosa* that someone could tolerate on their skin or in their nose becomes life-threatening when it enters your bloodstream.

But it's also not always about just the science. There are also broader social and economic factors that impact what is deemed newsworthy, and superbugs don't always fit the criteria. I mentioned that new problems are more likely to get our attention. But the story of superbugs is not new. It is nearly as old as antibiotics themselves. In fact, Alexander Fleming, the discoverer of penicillin, warned of the rise of antibiotic resistance in his Nobel Prize lecture in 1945:

> The time may come when penicillin can be bought by anyone in the shops. Then there is the danger that the ignorant man may easily underdose himself and by exposing his microbes to non-lethal quantities of the drug make them resistant. Here is a hypothetical illustration. Mr X has a sore throat. He buys some penicillin and gives himself, not enough to kill the streptococci but enough to educate them to resist penicillin. He then infects his wife. Mrs X gets pneumonia and is treated with penicillin. As the streptococci are now resistant to penicillin the treatment fails. Mrs X dies. Who is primarily responsible for Mrs X's death? Why Mr X whose negligent use of penicillin changed the nature of the microbe.
>
> *Moral:* If you use penicillin, use enough.

Today, that speech seems eerily prescient. But it also demonstrates the difficulty in getting the point across. The lay reader has to juggle with difficult concepts like resistance, antibiotics, and proper dosing!

Finally, there's also another reason the superbug pandemic remains hidden even in broad daylight. We cannot choose to ignore this if we are to effectively combat this threat. An issue that came to the fore during the COVID-19 pandemic is the disparity in global attention based on where deaths occur and who the victims are.

Antibiotic-resistant superbugs hit the youngest and the elderly the hardest. They are also prevalent in low-resource-healthcare settings and lower-income regions. Hospitals with sickly populations are hotbeds of superbug spread. Almost by definition, these populations have neither the loudest voices nor the fattest wallets: their deaths don't make international headlines.

A recurring theme in this book is that we will need to do a better job of treating antibiotics like a precious, shared resource. Here, a parallel can be drawn with our cavalier use of fossil fuels and how this has led to the climate crisis we currently face. The misuse of antibiotics has caused a similar superbug crisis in which those who are not responsible for the threat are the ones bearing the brunt of its impact.

However, as the COVID-19 pandemic has also shown, in our globalized world, pathogens – whether they're viruses or superbugs – don't respect borders. The challenges they pose aren't limited to just one region, they're a global problem. Just as the world united against COVID-19, it is imperative to face this microbial menace collectively. Understanding the imminent need for spreading awareness and adopting measures to deal with the threat, global leaders will convene under the aegis of the United Nations to discuss and strategize against this looming antibiotic resistance crisis in 2024. Investments in innovative solutions, from new antibiotics to effective vaccines and advanced diagnostic tools, are of paramount importance. But even simple acts like handwashing can go a long way in reducing the spread of infectious bacteria.

There's a bigger point that extends beyond superbugs. To think that we can conquer nature is a form of hubris with potentially disastrous consequences. From pandemics to climate change, this arrogance threatens not just individual lives, but also our collective well-being. To counteract this way of thinking, we must adopt a holistic approach, respecting the complexity and interconnectedness of the natural world we share with other forms of life.

3

Blindness in a Bottle

In early 2023, a chilling story unfolded across the US. Physicians were encountering patients with painfully inflamed eyes clouded by heavy yellow pus. These patients could sense light but were plunged into darkness. One doctor described a particular instance as the most severe eye infection he'd ever witnessed.

By piecing together these individual cases, scientists realized that these infections signalled the onset of a nationwide outbreak. By the time authorities sounded the alarm, fifty-eight Americans had been known to have been infected, five suffered permanent vision loss, and one tragically died.

The Centers for Disease Control and Prevention (CDC) in the US tracks disease outbreaks, while another government regulatory body, the Food and Drug Administration (FDA), approves drugs for treatment in that country. Now, the baton was passed on to the FDA, and their investigation brought them to India. All fingers pointed to a common source: contaminated eye drops. The culprit in the eye drops was found to be a formidable superbug.

Let's pause for a moment. Imagine going to the pharmacy and asking for something as innocuous as over-the-counter eye drops to moisten your eyes and a few days later suffering from a severe untreatable infection that had spread through your body. Imagine needing to have your eyeball removed to save your life. If there's a tragedy that epitomizes the interconnected and insidious nature of the hidden pandemic and how it has rudely entered our lives, it is this.

Connecting the dots in this case was no mean feat. Infected patients were spread across thirteen states, the timeline of their illnesses stretched over months, and the virulent superbug manifested in different parts of their bodies – from eyes to lungs to the bloodstream. It all began in May in Los Angeles county, California. Two patients were treated by the same ophthalmologist with severe eye infections. Soon after, two more cases emerged. Preliminary lab tests identified the culprit: a strain of *Pseudomonas aeruginosa*.

Here also is a key theme that underscores the silent nature of how superbugs have emerged and why they do not capture headlines like the emergence of a new virus such as the one that causes COVID-19. *Pseudomonas aeruginosa* is a common bacterium commonly found in many settings such as hospitals. You might even be harbouring strains of *Pseudomonas aeruginosa* right now on your skin, while feeling perfectly fine. But it's an opportunistic bacterium. In patients with compromised immune systems, wounds, or implanted medical devices, it can wreak havoc. If it infects blood or bone, then it can be potentially life-threatening for anyone.

Another thing that makes *Pseudomonas aeruginosa* hard to beat is that it can pick up the resistance genes that are the hallmark of superbugs. MDR *Pseudomonas aeruginosa*, which can defeat many antibiotics, is a leading cause of serious infections in healthcare settings. Around 13 per cent of *Pseudomonas aeruginosa* infections are MDR. That's what makes it one of our Deadly Six superbugs.

Pseudomonas aeruginosa typically spreads via contaminated medical equipment or hands. What set this outbreak apart was that it had spread through eye drops to the patients' eyes, a location where it's not commonly found. In addition, this specific superbug showcased resilience against everything physicians were throwing at it.

As the outbreak spread, genetic testing revealed that the infections across states were caused by a single previously unknown strain of *Pseudomonas aeruginosa*. Unfortunately, what the CDC had spotted was a set of supergenes in *Pseudomonas aeruginosa* that granted the superbug immunity against many common antibiotics. What this means was the strain contaminating the eye drops was worse than MDR: it was extremely-drug resistant (XDR) *Pseudomonas aeruginosa*.

> ## Penicillin Broken Down by Enzymes
> ## (Beta-Lactamases)
>
> [Chemical structure diagram of penicillin]
>
> **Image credit:** Wikipedia (public domain image)
>
> Penicillin is a kind of antibiotic known as a beta-lactam because of the presence of a ring, also called a beta-lactam (in light grey). Beta-lactam antibiotics include frequently prescribed drugs such as penicillins, cephalosporins, carbapenems, and monobactams. Beta-lactamases break down the beta-lactam ring, thus disarming the antibiotics.

This particular variant of *Pseudomonas aeruginosa* was impervious to common antibiotics, thanks to the production of two enzymes both encoded by resistance genes.

The superbug produced two enzymes known as beta-lactamases, which helped it fight against antibiotics. Unfortunately, beta-lactamase resistance genes are prevalent and spread readily. The proliferation of beta-lactamase resistance genes is a significant contributor to antibiotic resistance, complicating the treatment of bacterial infections.

The most prevalent types of beta-lactamases are classified based on their mechanism of action and structural characteristics. Some can neutralize a broad array of antibiotics, including advanced ones like carbapenems. Understanding these enzymes is critical for clinicians to select effective treatments and help curb the spread of resistance.

The two key enzymes that the deadly superbug made were Verona integron-encoded metallo-beta-lactamase (VIM) and Guiana-extended spectrum-beta-lactamase (GES).

VIM was first found in *Pseudomonas aeruginosa* isolated from a patient hospitalized at Verona University Hospital in northern Italy in 1997. VIM-producing superbugs are resistant to most antibiotics (including carbapenems) and can cause a wide range of infections, from urinary tract infections to sepsis. Since its discovery, VIM has spread widely across the world. There are over fifty known variants of VIM, each with potentially varying ability to inactivate antibiotics.

On the other hand, the GES enzyme was first reported from a strain of *Klebsiella pneumoniae* from an infant in French Guiana in 1998. GES can break down a broader spectrum of beta-lactam antibiotics, including penicillins and cephalosporins. To date, researchers have discovered over thirty variants of GES, indicating a diversifying arsenal that superbugs can employ to survive antibiotic treatment.

This superbug with a particular combination of VIM and GES in *Pseudomonas aeruginosa* had never been seen before in the US, and the CDC reported that it was resistant to at least twelve different antibiotic treatment options. Only one antibiotic was known to work against it in certain cases – cefiderocol.

At this point, all signs pointed towards a common product being the source. As the puzzle unravelled, the focus shifted to artificial tears. Most of the infected patients had used them. Investigations converged on a single product found across affected states manufactured by a Chennai-based company called Global Pharma Healthcare.

It was only after testing found that the bacteria was present in multiple bottles of the product that a public recall was issued. This recall subsequently expanded to other eyecare products from the same manufacturer.

By mid-May 2023, the CDC reported that the insidious strain had affected eighty-one individuals in eighteen states. These patients had been afflicted over the course of a year spanning May 2022 and April 2023. Their experiences with the superbug varied from unsettling vision issues to the need for enucleation (which is the surgical removal of the eye). And tragically, the outbreak resulted in four deaths.

Recognizing the mounting crisis, the FDA took decisive

action. They suspended the import of the implicated product and mandated an expansive recall. Yet, for many affected users, this response, while necessary, came as little solace. Consider the ordeal of Clara Elvira Oliva, a sixty-eight-year-old woman in Florida. For her, the encounter with this superbug was a deeply personal and devastating experience. Using the eye drops led to severe complications that culminated in the loss of her right eye.

Various concerns were voiced regarding the effectiveness of regulations in controlling imports of overseas medications, especially since the FDA had not inspected the Indian factory where the eye drops were produced before the outbreak had taken place. At the time, the frequency and quality of the FDA's inspections came under scrutiny, especially considering the significant drop in overseas inspections during the coronavirus pandemic. While the world's focus was on combating one health crisis, another had been brewing.

In fact, the FDA has long faced criticism for its inspection lapses, especially concerning overseas manufacturing units. Another criticism is that there were no mandatory inspections for producers of over-the-counter medicines, such as the infected eye drops, despite reports of contamination of drugs by other manufacturing units.

Upon closer inspection of the manufacturing unit, the lapse became evident. The FDA inspected the Indian plant between 20 February and 2 March 2023 unannounced, and they found several violations of practices with respect to sterility norms. Eleven of twenty-three bottles of eye drops that tested were found to be harbouring the bacteria, with seven of those directly matching the outbreak superbug.

Bloomberg reported that FDA inspectors found brown residue in the filling machines and improperly trained staff operating the plant. By this time, however, the manufacturer had shipped hundreds of thousands of bottles to the US without proper oversight, taking advantage of lax FDA rules and a largely unmonitored supply chain. And if this were not enough, neither the manufacturer nor the distributors had a substantial background in the US pharmaceutical industry.

Here's what should've happened. The sterile manufacturing of medical products, especially those used in sensitive areas like the eyes, should've followed an incredibly stringent protocol to the letter to ensure that the product remained free from harmful contaminants. And to ensure rules were followed, there should've been better oversight.

In a story published in the *New York Times* on 3 April 2023 Maroya Walters, lead investigator for the antimicrobial resistance team of the CDC, predicted: 'I think we are going to see the impact of this play out over the course of months to years.'

On 27 October, many months after the initial episode, the FDA issued the following warning on its website: 'The FDA is warning consumers not to purchase and to immediately stop using twenty-six over-the-counter eye drop products due to the potential risk of eye infections that could result in partial vision loss or blindness.'

At the time of writing in November 2023, the FDA was still expanding the list of eye drops that should not be purchased or used.

As tragic as these incidents are, they are only the tip of the iceberg. While the world dealt with the COVID-19 pandemic decisively, a quieter crisis has been brewing, and as I've said before, this crisis can potentially dwarf even the most catastrophic impacts of the COVID-19 pandemic.

Whether they originally come from human bodies or the environment, superbugs have developed sophisticated methods to combat antibiotics. They might change the parts of themselves that the drugs target, stop the antibiotics from entering, get rid of the antibiotics using special pumps, or even deactivate the antibiotics with specific enzymes. All these strategies combine to create a severe resistance problem that makes it very tough to treat infections caused by these superbugs with the antibiotics we have today.

Modern medical practice has resulted in an increase in the number of people with weaker immune systems. This group includes the very young, the elderly, those on medications that reduce immunity, and those with diseases that suppress their immune responses. Unfortunately, this has led to a rise in the infections caused by bacteria that naturally rise to the occasion.

More people need to be hospitalized, often for longer periods, exposing them to superbugs, especially in healthcare settings. Earlier, most of these resistant infections were linked to hospitals or other healthcare places where antibiotics were frequently used. Now, we're seeing resistant infections like MRSA coming from outside the healthcare system. Even more concerning is that some resistant bacteria, such as the penicillin-resistant *Streptococcus pneumoniae*, which often affects children, are mostly picked up in the community.

For an antibiotic to work properly, it has to stick to its intended target within the bacteria and interfere with the bacteria enough to stop its growth. This binding process is influenced by concentration of the antibiotic, its compatibility with the target, and time. Bacteria can resist antibiotics by controlling how much of the antibiotic gets inside and how much is pumped out.

Four of the Deadly Six superbugs, including resistant strains of *Pseudomonas aeruginosa* (like the one found in the eye drops), *Klebsiella pneumoniae*, *Acinetobacter baumannii*, and *E. coli* are designated as Gram-negatives to contrast them with other bacteria called Gram-positives.

This distinction is based on how we classify bacteria. Staining bacteria is a basic technique in microbiology that enhances the visibility of bacteria under a microscope. The Gram stain, specifically, is a differential staining method.

Bacteria that retain the crystal violet stain appear blue or violet (Gram-positive), while those that do not, and instead take up the counterstain appear red or pink (Gram-negative).

This distinction, which was first made by Danish microbiologist Hans Christian Gram (1853–1938) over a century ago, isn't just cosmetic. It categorizes bacteria based on the properties of their cell walls. Gram-positive bacteria have a thick layer that retains the violet dye, whereas Gram-negative bacteria have a thinner layer and an outer membrane that does not. This difference is clinically significant because it affects how bacteria interact with antibiotics and dictates how we approach treatment. So, the Gram stain is not only a diagnostic tool, it also guides antibiotic selection. For instance, penicillin is more effective against Gram-positive bacteria due to their cell wall structure.

The cell envelope of Gram-negative bacteria, on the other hand, has more intricate barriers that can naturally block the entry of many antibiotics. This complexity is why Gram-negative bacteria have been particularly worrying to physicians. The outer membrane of these bacteria is akin to an impenetrable shield that filters out unwanted substances. This membrane is less permeable than the cell walls of Gram-positive bacteria, making it much harder for antibiotics to get through. These bacteria also have structures called porins that work like gates and let small things in. While they do allow some substances to enter, they also block many antibiotics from passing through.

Just like medieval castles had walls and moats, bacterial cells have membranes studded with intricate structures that serve as the first line of defence. These structures can limit the entry of harmful agents, including antibiotics and toxins. Some bacteria even release bubble-like vesicles that act as decoys, attracting and neutralizing threats. In addition, Gram-negative bacteria possess an arsenal of biochemical tools to counteract the efforts of antibiotics. They produce enzymes, like the beta-lactamases we discussed, that can degrade or modify antibiotics to render them ineffective. In fact, many of the genes that get passed on to confer resistance give rise to enzymes readily in Gram-negative bacteria.

On the other hand, Gram-positive bacteria don't have this outer shield, and so they are often more vulnerable to antibiotics. However, some of them, like certain *Mycobacterium* species, have developed other ways to fend off the harmful effects of antibiotics.

The complexity of Gram-negative bacteria doesn't stop there. They are also equipped with efflux pumps. These are microscopic pumps that actively eject antibiotics and other unwanted chemicals from cells. They can be thought of as built-in waste management systems that can recognize and expel harmful substances. These pumps reduce the internal concentration of an antibiotic, making it less effective at its job.

Some bacteria, like *Pseudomonas aeruginosa*, which is found in diverse environments like soil and water, have an impressive array of these pumps. These mechanisms help bacteria adapt to varied surroundings and deal with threats like antibiotics.

Moreover, efflux pumps can have an environmental impact by raising the concentration of antibiotics in their vicinity. This can inhibit the growth of commensal bacteria, those that usually live in harmony with us, leading to a shift in the bacterial community composition. Within a few generations – this could be just days given the speed at which bacteria reproduce – more resistant bacteria can come to dominate, exacerbating the problem of antibiotic resistance.

All bacteria have genes that produce proteins responsible for moving small molecules in and out. Some pumps are like general cleaners, expelling a range of toxic substances and thus offering a natural resistance to antibiotics. But others are more specific. For instance, there is a pump designed mainly to get rid of tetracycline antibiotics. The activity of this pump is carefully regulated by another switch that ensures that it is used only when required.

The systems that control the movement of antibiotics are interconnected and influenced by a symphony of related proteins. When *E. coli* strains encounter antibiotics, they react in several ways. These bacteria turn on specific genes, alter parts of their outer layer, and adjust how they respond to stress. This results in general resistance in which the bacteria become resistant to multiple and different antibiotics.

However, other resistance strategies are more specific. Some bacteria produce enzymes that deactivate certain antibiotics. These enzymes can be very efficient. Some bacteria develop ways to bypass the effects of specific antibiotics, like the vancomycin antibiotic, with precision. Others alter their internal targets to avoid being affected by the antibiotics. For example, changes in certain genes can help bacteria resist antibiotics like fluoroquinolones or rifampin.

It's also worth pointing out that superbugs can use several different techniques to resist antibiotics all at the same time. For example, *Pseudomonas aeruginosa* uses a combination of methods to resist most aminoglycoside antibiotics. Also, it's not uncommon for bacteria to possess multiple resistance genes against different antibiotics as we saw in the case of the eye drop superbug. Managing such versatile resistance is a significant challenge.

Consider the enzymes that deactivate certain antibiotics. Many bacteria possess enzymes that target penicillin and similar antibiotics. While some of these resistance mechanisms are always 'on', others are triggered only in the presence of the antibiotic, providing protection just when needed.

One key strategy in the bacterial playbook for defeating antibiotics is to modify their targets through enzymes encoded by resistance genes. Many antibiotics work by attacking specific molecules in bacterial cells. Beta-lactam antibiotics like penicillin, for instance, attack enzymes responsible for building bacterial cell walls. However, some bacteria, such as MRSA, have modified enzymes that are no longer susceptible to these drugs. If an antibiotic is a key and its target is the lock, MRSA has changed the lock.

Bacteria have also developed other ways to nullify harmful substances before they can do damage. They do this by chemically modifying the substances or by producing special proteins that bind and neutralize them. It is as if bacteria have their own molecular 'bodyguards' that capture intruders before they can wreak havoc.

Interestingly, the bacteria that suffer damage can also repair themselves. Oxidative damage to bacterial DNA, which can be caused by exposure to antibiotics, is repaired through ancient and highly efficient systems. Some bacteria even have specialized enzymes that can mend their RNA, allowing them to recover from assaults that would otherwise be fatal.

Bacteria also have social protocols for defence. When a bacterial cell is attacked, it can release signals to warn its kin. *Bacillus subtilis*, for example, can modify its cell wall to hinder virus attachment when it senses a neighbouring cell is infected. Bacteria often operate as collectives, using what's known as 'quorum sensing' to evaluate their numbers. When they sense a high density of their kin, they expect an attack to be more likely and so they pre-emptively bolster defences.

Another common defensive tactic that relies on bacterial teamwork is the formation of biofilms, where they group together and produce a slimy, protective layer. This communal living arrangement makes it extremely hard for antibiotics to penetrate and kill the bacteria. As a result, biofilms can make bacterial infections more difficult to treat. Scientists think that breaking up biofilms can make bacteria more susceptible to antibiotics. And indeed, strategies such as the use of biofilm inhibitors can heighten the effectiveness of antibiotics, while lowering the chance for resistance to evolve.

Within bacterial populations, there's often a range of genetic variability. This means that some individuals might be more resistant to certain threats than others, providing an additional layer of protection for the community. Real-time damage is a reliable but often late indicator of a threat. Some bacteria are clever enough to sense danger before physical harm occurs by detecting chemical cues. For instance, they can eavesdrop on the communications between other strains to monitor their density and predict an upcoming assault.

In short, bacteria have evolved myriad different strategies to fend off antibiotics, whether by changing their protective outer layers, developing pumps to expel drugs, or altering their internal structures. They're also highly adaptable and capable of communicating with one another chemically to thwart antibiotics.

Understanding how bacteria develop resistance to antibiotics is a complex and somewhat disquieting task. However, grasping these details is essential for scientists and healthcare providers in their ongoing battle against superbug infections because we cannot fight what we do not understand.

4

The New Delhi Story

In 2010, an international group of scientists studying antibiotic resistance found themselves in the eye of a storm in India. The controversy was sparked by a paper they had published in *The Lancet Infectious Diseases*: 'Emergence of a New Antibiotic Resistance Mechanism in India, Pakistan and the UK: A Molecular, Biological and Epidemiological Study'. In this paper, they reported research on a gene conferring antibiotic resistance and commented that it was prevalent in patients in India and Pakistan. They claimed that from this epicentre, this supergene was spreading globally through superbugs that carried it.

Most scientific papers glide below the public's radar, attracting limited attention and scrutiny. They are downloaded and read only a few thousand times, mainly by specialists in the field. But that was not the case here. Within just two days of publication, the paper had amassed a staggering 4.7 million views online. The findings embroiled the authors in a socio-political storm. Questions arose, accusations flew, and the credibility and motivations of the scientists and the journal were questioned. This paper was also widely discussed on social media, and it was even brought up in the Indian parliament.

According to contemporaneous media reports, one of the authors disavowed some of the broader points in the discussion. The editor-in-chief of the parent journal, *The Lancet*, was reported to have apologized. Later, one of the lead authors claimed that his visa to India had been cancelled because of the fallout from the scientific paper. A decade later, while giving a talk on superbugs, he would describe the two years that followed the incident as 'toxic'.

What was all the fuss about? The paper mentioned an antibiotic resistance gene on a mobile element that hopped from one bacterial strain to another. Like other antibiotic genes, it contained the instructions to make an enzyme that could enable resistance to many antibiotics, turning carriers into superbugs. The enzyme belonged to the class we discussed earlier – beta-lactamases.

We should talk about the name of the gene and the enzyme: New Delhi metallo-beta-lactamase-1 or NDM-1. Much of the angst in India was because of the naming of the gene after New Delhi due to a purported connection with the nation's capital. The paper was published online in

The Lancet Infectious Diseases in August 2010 and collated in an issue in September. By October, media attention in India had moved on.

The ensuing debate over NDM-1 and its significance posed critical questions that were raised but never fully addressed in the broader public sphere at the time. In contrast, within the field of infectious diseases, that paper in *The Lancet Infectious Diseases* became a landmark. When scientists write research papers, they cite prior relevant work in the reference sections. How many times a paper is cited is a useful metric to gauge its importance. In 2021, an editorial in *The Lancet Infectious Diseases* mentioned that the NDM-1 antibiotic resistance paper published in 2010 had received the fourth-highest number of citations among all papers published during the journal's twenty years of continuous publication. In a little over a decade, the paper had been cited by over 2,000 other scientific papers.

You might be curious about what the most-cited paper in the journal was. That paper too dealt with antibiotic resistance, highlighting the significance of superbugs. But that threat would come later from China, and we will get to that too. But first, let's look at NDM-1.

To unravel the full story, we must look back to a time before the paper in *The Lancet Infectious Diseases* created a furore. This paper wasn't the first instance of this gene being reported, and nor was it the first documented report in which the gene's origin was tied to New Delhi. In fact, the discovery of the resistance gene and its naming after New Delhi had been documented in a scientific paper called 'Characterization of a New Metallo-β-Lactamase Gene, blaNDM-1, and a Novel Erythromycin Esterase Gene Carried on a Unique Genetic Structure in *Klebsiella pneumoniae* Sequence Type 14 from India' published in 2009 in another journal called *Antimicrobial Agents and Chemotherapy*. The ordeal of just one patient mentioned in the paper would unexpectedly ignite a maelstrom. Neither the patient nor the authors of that first paper could have foreseen the havoc they would unleash.

The 2009 research paper starts with the medical history of a fifty-nine-year-old man. Here's what we know about him. He was originally from India, but he settled in Sweden for many years and frequently travelled back to his native country. From his medical history, we know he had diabetes and that he had suffered multiple strokes. We don't know his name, but from the medical records of this 'Swedish patient of Indian origin', there's nothing remarkable about his earlier trips to India.

However, a visit to India in November 2007 marked the start of a precarious medical odyssey. Within a month, the man found himself admitted to a hospital in Ludhiana, Punjab, due to a significant gluteal abscess, or a collection of pus in the area of his buttocks resulting from an infection. Soon after, he underwent surgery at a New Delhi hospital where, to complicate matters, he developed a bedsore. During his medical treatments, he was exposed to a battery

The New Delhi Story

of potent antibiotics, including amoxicillin-clavulanic acid and amikacin.

Upon the man's return to Sweden, a clearer picture of his torment began to emerge. The medical team in Örebro, Sweden, identified a bacterial strain of *Klebsiella pneumoniae* in the man's urine, even though he had shown no signs of a urinary tract infection. We should recall here that *Klebsiella pneumoniae* is one of our Deadly Six superbugs.

Physicians also discovered another concerning presence: a superbug variant of *E. coli* that produced extended spectrum beta-lactamases in the man's faeces. This is also one of the Deadly Six superbugs. *E. coli* can coexist within and with us harmlessly, but its variants that cause disease and produce antibiotic-breaking enzymes from resistance genes have the alarming capability of thwarting common antibiotics, making them formidable clinical adversaries.

A deeper dive into the biological signatures of these two superbugs yielded more disturbing findings. The *K. pneumoniae* strain showed resistance to carbapenems. Both this superbug and the isolated *E. coli* superbug were resistant to most beta-lactams. Here's where the plot thickened. Despite their intensive search, the scientists couldn't find any known antibiotic resistance genes. They were facing a scientific mystery. Was it possible that the superbug had a completely new resistance gene that science had not yet discovered?

Determined to get to the bottom of this, the scientists

decided to investigate further. They theorized that if the superbug was not exhibiting resistance due to any known genes, it must have a novel gene causing this resilience. To uncover this mysterious gene, they embarked on an extensive exploration. They constructed a genomic library – essentially a collection of all the genes present in the superbug. Thus, they aimed to isolate and test each gene to see which one was providing *E. coli* the antibiotic resistance.

Their perseverance paid off when they identified a previously undiscovered gene responsible for the superbug's ability to fend off antibiotics. This gene gave rise to a new kind of beta-lactamase enzyme.

Naming conventions in microbiology are often systematic, reflecting certain characteristics or origins of the discovery. Following this tradition, the scientists named the new gene 'New Delhi metallo-beta-lactamase-1'. The name had a twofold significance. 'New Delhi' was chosen as a prefix because it was believed that the patient might have acquired the infection during a visit to New Delhi. Recall from the previous chapter how other beta-lactamase genes are named after Verona in Italy and French Guiana. The latter part of the name, 'metallo-beta-lactamase', describes the function of the enzyme produced by the gene. This enzyme specifically targets and breaks down a group of antibiotics known as beta-lactams (described in the previous chapter).

But let's be very clear, New Delhi metallo-beta-lactamase-1, or NDM-1, isn't an organism, or even a gene. It is an enzyme encoded by a particular gene which we will call the NDM-1 gene for the sake of clarity.

This gene (NDM-1) gives rise to an enzyme that troubled scientists because it was an effective defence against a broad range of beta-lactam antibiotics. It was particularly adept at neutralizing antibiotics like penicillin and cephalosporins. Worryingly, bacteria carrying the NDM-1 gene were also resistant to carbapenems, which are a critical class of antibiotics often used to treat MDR infections. Therefore, infections caused by superbugs harbouring NDM-1 would be challenging to treat, leading to an increased likelihood of prolonged hospital stays and death.

The NDM-1 gene was part of a mobile genetic element that could move from one bacterial species to another, like from *Klebsiella pneumoniae* to *E. coli*. This mobility allows the gene to spread resistance traits between different types of bacteria. The transportation mechanism was plasmids, which, as we have discussed earlier, are small snippets of DNA that facilitate gene transfers between bacteria.

Not only was the gene worrying, but now the researchers also knew that it was transferred effectively among bacteria. This mechanism transformed an ordinary bacterium into a superbug resistant to most known antibiotics of our time. It's this transference capability of the gene, particularly through plasmids, that was a worrying omen for potential spread.

We should take a small detour and talk about resistance genes and what they actually do. NDM-1 is a gene that acts as a blueprint for bacteria to make an enzyme called a carbapenemase. The '-ase' addition indicates that this enzyme can accelerate chemical reactions that break apart carbapenems. But carbapenemases have an extensive 'toolkit' that allows them to break down many antibiotics apart from carbapenems. This makes them particularly dangerous because they don't just resist one type of drug – they can resist several.

The history of these antibiotic-resistant genes goes back to the early 1990s, to Japan where bacteria started to display resistance to a group of antibiotics called carbapenems. The first gene and enzyme identified that neutralized carbapenems was called IMP-1, and this too was found on a plasmid.

Shortly after the identification of IMP-1, a different type of resistance gene was discovered, VIM-1. The acronym 'VIM' stands for 'Verona Integron-encoded Metallo-beta-lactamase'. This name is derived from the city of Verona in Italy, famously known as the setting of several Shakespeare plays, including *Romeo and Juliet*.

VIM-1 is a type of enzyme that confers resistance to certain antibiotics, particularly to those in the beta-lactam class – just like IMP-1. The discovery of VIM-1 in Verona highlights the ongoing global emergence of antibiotic resistance genes.

The global implications of these resistant strains became even more apparent when, in 1996, a strain of *Klebsiella pneumoniae* resistant to carbapenems emerged in the US.

Unlike the IMP-1 and VIM-1 enzymes, this strain produced a previously unknown enzyme that researchers named KPC, an abbreviation of *Klebsiella pneumoniae* carbapenemase.

The *Antimicrobial Agents Chemotherapy* research article was the first warning that a new global threat was emerging. Though the findings were significant for infectious disease researchers, this paper escaped the attention of the Indian public. First, it was a report of a new resistance gene in one patient who had specific challenges with his health. Second, it wasn't the first gene ever identified that broke down carbapenem antibiotics. Third, there was no smoking gun showing that the gene had widely spread across bacteria present in human populations.

This information is important to put NDM-1 in the right context. While the discovery and spread of NDM-1 caused concern, we should note that its discovery is different from finding a new virus like the coronavirus that caused COVID-19. NDM-1 wasn't the first carbapenemase to be identified, and given the propensity for resistance genes to be shared, it very likely won't be the last. However, the researchers ended the 2009 paper with a warning. 'In a country where there is little control on antibiotic prescriptions, the rapid dissemination of such a plasmid is alarming.'

This warning would soon turn out to be prescient. Later in 2009, a team of researchers at P.D. Hinduja National Hospital and Medical Research Centre in Mumbai found twenty-four strains of bacteria that were resistant to carbapenems. Of these, twenty-two were producing the NDM-1 enzyme. Most of these were strains of *Klebsiella* and *E. coli*, but researchers also found three other bacterial species. Within one part of India at least, the resistance gene seemed to be spreading. This report, titled 'New Delhi Metallo-Beta Lactamase (NDM-1) in Enterobacteriaceae: Treatment Options with Carbapenems Compromised', which was published in the *Journal of the Association of Physicians of India*, also flew under the radar.

That would all change in 2010 with the paper in *The Lancet Infectious Diseases*. We were no longer dealing with just one patient or even one city. This paper identified multiple people dealing with the NDM-1 resistance genes, and it explicitly pointed to India and Pakistan as the hub of an emerging superbug crisis.

The research paper painted a vivid picture of a landscape in which resistance genes could hitch rides across continents, hidden in the DNA of bacteria, aided by human travel and migration. To emphasize the urgency of the threat, the paper also cited a past resistance gene first detected in India during the mid-1990s, which had rapidly achieved global prevalence.

A focal point of concern was the rising resistance in Gram-negative bacteria. For the reasons discussed in the preceding chapter, crafting antibiotics to combat these bacteria has been challenging. As a result, carbapenems had emerged as a beacon of hope, often considered the last line of defence. But with NDM-1 joining other resistance genes in threatening their efficacy, the authors sounded a dire warning.

Superbugs possessing the NDM-1 gene demonstrated formidable antibiotic resistance. In the UK, samples resisted key antibiotics like imipenem, ertapenem, and aztreonam. Superbugs from the city of Chennai in India displayed resistance to a gamut of antibiotics, including beta-lactam antibiotics, fluoroquinolones, and aminoglycosides. Treatment options were increasingly limited.

The researchers noted the presence of the NDM-1 gene across various-sized mobile plasmids in different bacteria, implying the gene's ability to shuttle effortlessly between bacterial hosts, which further deepened the concern. Alarmingly, some samples even exhibited multiple copies of the NDM-1 gene, either integrated within their primary DNA or on transferable plasmids. The gene was clearly hopping around and showing up in places where we least expected to find it.

That research paper published in 2010 also highlighted the global nature of this threat. Bacteria equipped with the NDM-1 gene were identified not only in various cities in India and Pakistan, but also in people with travel history linked to the subcontinent. The research paper suggested that we weren't dealing with a regional issue – it had global ramifications. Given the gene's high global mobility rate, the ease of resistance spread among bacteria became a glaring worry.

The publication of the research paper in *The Lancet Infectious Diseases* also ignited wider controversy. Let's take a closer look at some of the points it raised and critique them. Having laid out the scientific findings, we can examine them and consider their broader implications.

In hindsight, I think the most vociferous criticisms of the paper stemmed from three concerns that are all worth dissecting in detail.

The first concern was that the name stigmatized (or worse, blamed) India and its capital city for causing the spread of antibiotic-resistant genes. The words 'New Delhi' were in the name itself! The second concern was that the paper placed an undue emphasis on weaknesses in India's medical scenario that enabled the spread of superbugs. The third concern was with comments in the discussion section of the paper linking elective surgeries to the possible spread of this antibiotic resistance gene.

It would help here to explain the structure of a standard scientific article. It is typically structured to answer questions in a logical format. The introduction sets the stage by laying out what is already known. The experimental section deals with what the researchers of the current work actually did. The results elaborate on what they found, and the conclusion and discussion sections elaborate on the significance of the findings, any known limitations, and directions for future studies. It's not unusual, but indeed expected, that authors will expand on the implications of their studies in future research.

The New Delhi Story

I believe that the view that *The Lancet Infectious Diseases* article had cast India in the role of a primary culprit for the NDM-1 outbreak was at the heart of the political discontent in India in 2010. Some commentators even assigned the authors ulterior motives, stating that it was an orchestrated attempt by Western detractors to tarnish India's image and destabilize its economic standing. For example, angry members of Parliament in India questioned the study, saying it was funded by multinational pharmaceutical companies.

The reality is more complex. One of the authors declared that they had received a travel grant from a pharmaceutical company, and another declared they had commercial interests in a few listed companies. However, this type of declaration is common in biomedical research, and authors are expected to make these disclosures when they submit their articles. The research itself was not funded by pharmaceutical companies, but through grants from the European Union and the Wellcome Trust, a charitable institution. As far as I could tell, everything seemed above board here.

Then there was the issue of the name. According to multiple media outlets, in 2011, Richard Horton, the editor-in-chief of the parent journal, *The Lancet*, had confessed that naming the gene after New Delhi unfairly stigmatized India, saying, 'It was an error of judgement ... We didn't think of its implications for which I sincerely apologize,' while adding that the name should be changed.

I agree with Horton that it would have been better to

have not named the gene after New Delhi, but I'll get to that. But the mea culpa is puzzling for three reasons. First, as we just discussed, the naming of the gene had occurred prior to the controversy in 2010 and had nothing to do with *The Lancet Infectious Diseases* paper. Second, Horton is the editor-in-chief of *The Lancet* and not *The Lancet Infectious Diseases* journal. It is unlikely that he would have known of the 2010 research article when it was submitted. Third, since the journals are editorially independent, even if he knew and the gene had not been named yet, changing the name would not have been expected to be within his purview as editor of a separate journal.

What about the others involved in the process of publication? The research article in *The Lancet Infectious Diseases* was peer reviewed, and the reviewers would have certainly offered comments to the editor and the authors. The authors would also have needed to address these comments to the satisfaction of the editor prior to acceptance. But editors of scientific journals do not unilaterally name or change the name of key discoveries. That would cross the line into authorship. Also, their expertise lies in scrutinizing publications for scientific accuracy rather than in addressing political sensitivities relating to nomenclature.

But what about the name of the gene itself? In the world of scientific discovery, naming conventions have an essential role. They not only offer a way to identify and categorize discoveries, but in some cases, they provide insights into their origin or characteristics. Naming the gene 'NDM-1' may have been meant as a marker for first identification to distinguish it from other resistance genes without any intent to cause hurt. This naming choice was not a first-of-its-kind decision. Instead, it was in line with established microbiological conventions. Just as resistance genes have been named after places like São Paulo in Brazil and Verona in Italy, NDM-1 was named after New Delhi following an established convention.

There is a distinction between naming resistance genes and the WHO's recommendations on naming viruses and pathogens. The WHO advises against associating viruses with specific locations to avoid potential stigmatization and misconceptions. The rationale behind this is clear: naming a virus after a place can inadvertently give the location negative connotations, leading to misinformation and prejudice. The WHO is absolutely right in this regard. However, there is no such advisory against naming resistance genes after locations.

I think it would be worth it in a socio-political context if microbiologists had a robust, nuanced debate on this matter. In the most recent past, the global pandemic caused by the novel coronavirus highlighted the sensitivities around the naming of diseases and their pathogens. It became widely accepted that the virus that caused the pandemic should be referred to as 'SARS-CoV-2' instead of the 'Wuhan virus' to avoid stigmatizing the city where it was first discovered. This naming decision was more than just semantics – it recognized the potential harm in associating a global health crisis with a specific location.

In this light, it's understandable why naming a resistance gene 'NDM-1' after New Delhi is problematic. Even if the discoverers were following established conventions, associating a city with a gene that can turn bacteria into deadly superbugs painted a negative picture of New Delhi and India. Such naming choices can perpetuate stereotypes or biases, even if unintentionally.

In the post-COVID-19 world, where the significance of names has become even more pronounced, it's crucial for the scientific community to approach naming with a sense of responsibility, ensuring that names serve a purpose without casting blame. The debate around the term 'NDM-1' serves as a reminder of the broader implications of scientific nomenclature. It underscores the need for a more thoughtful approach, one that takes into consideration not only the conventions of the past but has also an evolving understanding of the present. Scientists must recognize the impact of naming decisions, not just within their research communities but within society at large.

It is also important to note the stance of the Indian health ministry on this matter. They highlighted that the resistance gene isn't exclusive to any particular region. Instead, it can be found 'in the environment, and potentially in the intestines of both humans and animals'. While this may seem alarming, it is probably true. Contrary to popular opinion, resistance to natural antibiotics is a natural phenomenon. Indeed, long before humans started harnessing the power of antibiotics, microbes in the environment were already producing them. As a natural countermeasure, other microbes evolved and developed mechanisms to resist these antibiotics.

However, the central issue is the role of human actions in this equation. While antibiotic resistance is a natural phenomenon, human practices have significantly accelerated its spread. The 2010 research article in *The Lancet Infectious Diseases* foregrounded this very concern. The misuse and overuse of antibiotics, especially in places where they are readily available without prescriptions, can only exacerbate the situation. In essence, while antibiotic resistance is a part of the natural order of things, human interventions have amplified its reach and speed. Recognizing and addressing these human-induced factors is essential in our global fight against superbugs.

Wherever diseases are rampant and antibiotics are used without medical oversight, conditions are ripe for superbugs to thrive and for resistance to spread. These conditions are not unique to India, but the country was at the centre of this particular storm. We cannot be sure where the antibiotic resistance gene originated, but it was likely spreading for a while before it was identified.

Another point to remember is while NDM-1 was unique in many respects, it was not the first carbapenem antibiotic resistance gene identified or the only one of note. Nor was

India the only country where this type of resistance had been identified. The history of similar resistance genes and enzymes that move from one bacterium to another goes back to the 1990s. Superbugs had been identified with these genes in places like New York, Japan, and Italy.

A perspective published in the leading medical journal the *New England Journal of Medicine* in 2010 stated, 'Thus far, the majority of isolates in countries throughout the world can be traced to subjects who have travelled to India to visit family or have received medical care there. However, the ability of this genetic element to spread rapidly . . . means that there will almost certainly be numerous secondary cases throughout the world that are unrelated to travel to the Indian subcontinent.' Tourism and, more specifically, medical tourism, play a significant role in the global economy, with countries like India leading the way. India has become a top destination for medical tourism because of its ability to provide excellent medical care at a fraction of the cost of Western countries.

The 2010 paper in *The Lancet Infectious Diseases* had caused great concern when it hinted that this booming industry might inadvertently contribute to the global spread of the NDM-1 resistance gene. The paper suggested that international patients, travelling to India for medical care, could unintentionally carry this resistance back to their home countries. This suggestion in the paper in the discussion section caused quite an uproar. In fact, the backlash was so intense that one of the authors of the paper allegedly felt the need to distance themselves from this specific claim.

Admittedly, this is a delicate topic, with potential implications for a country's reputation and economy. However, the opinion was stated in the discussion section of a scientific article by researchers commenting broadly on the implications of their work. It's necessary for us to remember and separate actual results from informed perspectives on implications.

The backlash was unnecessary. Scientists should be free to offer their thoughts on their own research even if we disagree with their views. Science is self-correcting, but it thrives on debate and discussion. Haranguing scientists who make important contributions with public health implications or impugning their motives may help to support a political standpoint, but science suffers in the process.

Health officials responded by emphasizing that infections carrying the NDM-1 resistance gene could be managed and prevented with robust infection-control measures, a standard practice in any reputable hospital. Their confidence in the healthcare system's ability to manage such threats was also echoed by the CDC in the US.

However, not everyone shared this optimism. The author of the aforementioned *New England Journal of Medicine* perspective, for instance, had a more cautious point of view. He referenced historical patterns to suggest that while immediate solutions might seem effective, they might not be the final answer to such challenges, even in well-developed healthcare systems. Antibiotic resistance genes spread too easily, the threat of superbugs is too great, and our track record in combating spread leaves much to be desired.

The debate around the scientific article highlighted the complex interplay between science, public health, economy and international relations. But a key question remained: what would happen next?

In 2011, the next chapter of the saga unfolded and that was covered in *The Lancet Infectious Diseases* journal as well. A new research paper entitled 'Dissemination of NDM-1 Positive Bacteria in the New Delhi Environment and Its Implications for Human Health: An Environmental Point Prevalence Study' unveiled that the superbug-causing gene, NDM-1, wasn't just confined to hospitals. It had now been detected in public drinking water and street runoff in New Delhi. This meant that the threat was now lurking in everyday environments, turning public areas into potential hotspots for the spread of the resistance gene.

To understand the scale of the issue, scientists took a systematic approach. They collected water samples from various spots in and around New Delhi, focusing on a twelve-kilometre radius from the city centre. This effort included samples from street runoff and public tap water, and the results were concerning. Out of fifty drinking water samples, two tested positive for the NDM-1 gene. What was even more distressing was that the gene was found in 51 out of

171 street runoff samples. The fact that these contaminated sources were located in densely populated parts of the city added to the gravity of the situation.

But the challenges didn't end there. As researchers delved deeper, they found that the NDM-1 gene had made its way into bacterial species that it hadn't been previously linked to. This included bacteria like *Shigella boydii* and *Vibrio cholerae*. *Shigella boydii* is a bacterial species that causes shigellosis, or bacillary dysentery, characterized by diarrhoea (which can be bloody) along with fever and stomach cramps. *Vibrio cholerae*, on the other hand, is responsible for causing cholera. The ability of the gene to infiltrate various bacterial species highlighted its adaptability and resilience.

The implications of these findings were clear and worrying. With the NDM-1 bacteria being found in the city's environmental samples, it now posed a significant health threat. The city's vast population, many of whom depended on shared water sources and public sanitation facilities, were at increased risk. This wasn't just a health issue any more – it was also an infrastructural and societal challenge.

Soon, superbugs carrying the NDM-1 gene were becoming a major concern worldwide. Within a few years after they were first identified, they were found in numerous countries – Bangladesh, Pakistan, the US, the UK, Israel, Turkey, China, Australia, France, Japan, Kenya, Singapore, Taiwan and the Netherlands. The list of countries recognizing the presence of these superbugs was long, and it was growing. And that was only the tip of the iceberg. Since there wasn't a standard test available to detect the gene, many more countries likely had superbugs harbouring NDM-1 without even knowing it.

By 2017, things took another twist. Scientists found that the NDM-1 gene wasn't the only version out there. They discovered several variations of this gene, with some differing only slightly from the original. Some of these variants resulted in only one or a few changes in the make-up of the antibiotic-destroying enzyme. Interestingly, most of these NDM-1 superbugs seemed to have a strong presence in Asia, particularly in China and India. And it wasn't just people who were affected. The gene was also found in bacteria from animals. This raised a concerning possibility: these superbugs could be spreading through the food chain.

This brings us to 2023. A report in the scientific journal *PLoS Medicine* shed light on a worrying trend. The leading cause of newborn infections worldwide, *Klebsiella pneumoniae*, has developed a powerful defence against carbapenem. This study, which gathered data from thirty countries, found that a small but significant percentage of these infections in newborns in hospitals were caused by the carbapenem-resistant *Klebsiella* superbug. Alarmingly, nearly a quarter of these newborns didn't survive the infection.

To be clear, NDM-1 was not the only gene that led to superbugs resistant to carbapenems, but its emergence and spread caused great concern because it had a knack for moving quickly between different types of bacteria and spreading to different parts of the world. To make matters worse, without standard tests to spot it, many people were likely carrying superbugs without even knowing it. NDM-1 containing bacteria were also hard to defeat. For example, *E. coli* with NDM-1 caused complications from urinary tract infections to life-threatening conditions like sepsis. With limited effective antibiotics available, treatment becomes notably challenging.

However, in this looming darkness, there was a glimmer of hope from an unexpected source – an old antibiotic. Once sidelined due to its side effects, this medicine was now being revisited as a potential weapon against these relentless superbugs.

5

The Last Line Falls

It's estimated that hundreds of millions of residents in the Indian subcontinent carry superbugs in their gut that exhibit resistance to the class of antibiotics known as carbapenems. In the gut, these bacteria typically don't cause any problems, but if they spread and cause infection in other parts of the body, carbapenems won't work against them.

When carbapenems fell to resistant superbugs, it was a crisis. But there was still hope left for humanity in the form of an antibiotic which had fallen out of favour because it was considered too toxic to use. An antibiotic from the late 1950s, colistin was originally discovered in Japan from the soil bacterium *Bacillus polymyxa*. Colistin began to be used there and in Europe as an intravenous treatment. By 1959, the FDA had recognized its effectiveness against Gram-negative bacteria, and approved it for treating a range of infections, including diarrhoeal diseases and urinary tract infections. Such an expansive antibiotic range made colistin invaluable, especially when it was discovered that it could act against multi-resistant strains of *Pseudomonas aeruginosa*, which was then a significant medical challenge.

However, colistin's initial promise was marred by toxicity. It causes serious kidney damage and even affects the brain. Because our kidneys help remove toxic substances from our bodies, doctors must be careful with how much of the drug they administer. I've heard physicians call colistin a 'detergent', and it's not far from the truth.

Just as detergent removes grease and dirt from dishes, colistin disrupts the protective outer layer of bacterial cells. However, scientists were puzzled about how exactly colistin managed to 'clean away' Gram-negative bacteria and lead to their death. More than seven decades after the discovery of colistin, in a paper published in the *eLife* journal in 2021, researchers found that it targets a special ingredient inside bacteria such as *E. coli*.

The use of colistin was monitored over time and as other safer antibiotics were discovered, it was relegated to the back of the global medicine cabinet. After that, colistin was mostly used just for eye conditions and skin treatments. It was also given to patients with cystic fibrosis, either intravenously or as a mist they could inhale.

But with the lengthening shadow of superbugs resistant to carbapenems, physicians had no choice but to return to colistin. Colistin was revisited as a last-chance option to treat tenacious, MDR superbug infections.

Pseudomonas infections are amongst the most common, picked up in hospital stays of a week or more, and physicians tend to use colistin to treat them. They are also using colistin to treat infections caused by other superbugs from the Deadly Six as well like *Acinetobacter*, *E. coli*, and *Klebsiella pneumoniae*.

But let's make one thing clear. The resurgence of colistin in medicine isn't a sign of progress, it is a sign of desperation. The very fact that we need to go back to an antibiotic that was once shelved because of its toxicity highlights the dire situation in the battle against antibiotic resistance.

Colistin resistance has not developed partly because it had not been used extensively in humans. But in the shadows, colistin was being used in agriculture, and you probably have an inkling of what happened next. Before 2015, there were only a few rare cases where bacteria displayed resistance to colistin. But when these bacteria reproduced, they passed this resistance vertically through their chromosomal DNA to their descendants. As with other superbugs, the greatest concern arises when resistance genes can be spread even more rapidly through mobile elements like plasmids.

Soon enough, scientists noticed an unsettling trend: more and more bacteria isolated from animals in China were becoming resistant to colistin. In late 2015, the medical community was taken aback by a breathtaking discovery. A new resistance gene was identified in a pig in China, and it was named MCR-1, which stands for Mobile Colistin Resistance-1. The discovery was published in *The Lancet Infectious Diseases*. I mentioned in Chapter 4 how the discovery of NDM-1 was one of the most highly cited papers in *The Lancet Infectious Diseases*. It was surpassed by the discovery of MCR-1, which, by 2021, had become the most cited paper in the journal's history.

What makes MCR-1 particularly alarming is that like NDM-1, it is found on a plasmid, a mobile piece of DNA. This mobility allows the gene to be transferred easily between bacteria, offering a pathway for rapid spread of resistance.

The MCR-1 gene was found in *E. coli* taken from animals meant for human consumption in China. Between 2011 and 2014, in China, 15 per cent of raw meat samples, 21 per cent of animals and even 1 per cent of hospital patients with infections had the MCR-1 gene. Such widespread presence of the gene painted a grim picture.

By 2017, research by various scientists had delved deeper into the presence and impact of MCR-1 in China, and the results were concerning. Certain populations, notably males and individuals with compromised immune systems, were particularly susceptible. The study also found a strong link between the occurrence of the MCR-1 gene and previous antibiotic use. However, what stood out most was the rate at which the gene was being shared between bacteria. MCR-1 was hopping across different types of plasmids and into various strains of *E. coli* at an alarming frequency. This high transferability signified that MCR-1 had the potential to spread far and wide, making containing it even more challenging if not impossible.

Piecing these findings together, it became evident that superbugs resistant to colistin had infiltrated various regions of China. And sure enough, in a short time, MCR-1 was identified in bacteria in the US and then in other countries, sounding alarm bells in the global health community.

This highlights another significant aspect of the spread of antibiotic resistance, which is the extensive use of antibiotics globally to promote growth in livestock, especially animals raised for food. While some countries had already stopped using colistin for livestock, some major players in the global market, like China and India, continued this practice.

Soon, MCR-1 wasn't just found in hospitals; it was turning up in all kinds of places, from rivers in China to beaches in Brazil. A 2018 study revealed a global picture, tracing the explosive spread of MCR-1 back to one event that took place around 2006. Researchers used a powerful tool called whole-genome sequencing to track down the history of this potent gene. They found traces of a genetic event that set off a chain reaction, allowing the gene to spread far and wide. The gene moved between bacteria in transposons and got inserted into plasmids (we discussed both mobile elements in Chapter 2). This mobility was crucial to its subsequent spread.

Interestingly, this spread seemed to have begun with

livestock in China, highlighting how farms and agriculture might be playing a part in spreading antibiotic resistance.

Further studies have added more layers to this narrative. In 2022, a comprehensive analysis scanned a vast amount of genetic data, identifying not just the spread of MCR-1 but other descendants of MCR too with genetic modifications. Some of these resistance genes have been around longer than we thought, silently present in the environment for years before they caught the scientific world's attention.

The discovery of the MCR-1 gene was especially alarming for the global health community because it signified that superbugs had found a way to resist the last line of defence in antibiotics. So, let's step back and consider the implications of this. If a superbug which is already resistant to other antibiotics acquires MCR-1, it also becomes resistant to colistin, rendering the entire human antibiotic arsenal ineffective against it. This is not difficult to imagine since bacteria have the propensity to pick up more than one resistance gene in the process of becoming superbugs.

In China, because of the high prevalence of MCR-1 gene in livestock, it's quite possible that the use of colistin has unintentionally paved the way for the evolution of resistant bacteria no longer affected by the antibiotic. As a result, humans were being exposed to these superbugs either directly or by consuming meat from treated animals. The situation is further complicated by the fact that many other countries are recording increasing rates of colistin resistance. This is happening simultaneously because the rise of superbugs has led to a surge in the use of colistin in human medicine.

A detailed analysis in the journal *Pathogens* from studies conducted worldwide published from December 2014 to March 2021 painted a fuller picture of the spread of MCR-1. This investigation found that over 6 per cent of *E. coli* worldwide had developed resistance to the antibiotic colistin due to MCR genes. Worryingly, this resistant strain was found spread across fifty-four countries spanning five continents. A notable discovery was that chickens and pigs were the main carriers of this superbug.

If resistance spreads unchecked across different Gram-negative superbugs, we could face a situation in which many infections suddenly become untreatable. It seems like a doomsday scenario, but it is actually not far off from where we are today. That's why countries like India are undergoing massive surveillance of health data and data sharing to gauge the spread of resistance.

Fortunately, both China and India acted responsibly after the danger became known. The discovery of colistin-resistant superbugs with the MCR-1 gene led to immediate and comprehensive discussions among the scientific community. By April 2017, China had significantly reduced the production of colistin and had banned its use as an additive for promoting growth in animals.

With China banning the use of colistin, the focus turned on India. The country's rapidly growing poultry industry hid a fact from most consumers – antibiotics are used widely to boost growth in birds. This is the norm in many other countries as well, but in 2018, colistin was one of the antibiotics in use in India. An investigative report brought to light the unsettling fact that this crucial antibiotic was being freely used in the country's poultry sector, greatly undermining its essential role in healthcare.

India was spurred into action and in July 2019, in a landmark move, the Indian government banned the use of colistin in agriculture. To the credit of India's health ministry, the notification was strongly worded, and it expressly prohibited the 'manufacture, sale, and distribution of colistin and its formulations' for all food-producing animals, in poultry, in aquaculture, or even as supplements in animal feed. This is one of the strongest bans on the use of colistin in effect in the world.

The groundwork for this ban was laid by recommendations from India's premier drug advisory entity, the Drugs Technical Advisory Board and the National Antimicrobial Resistance Action Plan committee. These endorsements found momentum when a Bombay High Court case cited evidence highlighting the widespread misuse of colistin in Indian farming. This revelation propelled legal advocates to seek a ban on the over-the-counter sale of antibiotics for livestock. In essence, India's ban on colistin in farming demonstrated the willingness of the government to act quickly and decisively. The task now is to ensure the effective implementation of the ban.

The Last Line Falls

What broad lessons can we draw from this string of events? The existence of resistance genes to every major antibiotic is a testament to the adaptability of microbes. In the vast genetic repository of the natural world, these genes have been lying dormant, waiting for their moment. The vectors of their spread are primarily mobile genetic elements, such as plasmids, that facilitate the horizontal transfer of resistance genes between bacterial populations.

As these genes proliferate, antibiotics that were once pillars of modern medicine, considered unfailingly reliable, begin to falter. However, this isn't a new story nor will this be the last chapter of this saga.

One of the pivotal strategies in our adaptive response is the judicious use of antibiotics. We must begin to think of them not as commonplace drugs but as invaluable resources to be deployed sparingly at need. Their misuse and overuse, both in the medical sphere and in agricultural practices, can inadvertently expedite the emergence of superbugs. By narrowing their use to essential cases, we can extend the lifespan of these drugs, preserving their efficacy and delaying the emergence of resistant strains. This more conservative approach doesn't just preserve the power of our current antibiotics, but it also provides the scientific community with precious time to research, innovate, and develop new antibiotics or alternative treatments.

Saving lives is at the core of this strategy. By safeguarding the potency of our antibiotics and using them judiciously, we give patients the best chance of recovery when these drugs are truly needed. It's a paradigm shift in how we think about and use these drugs – a shift from wastefulness to conservation.

In 2016, after MCR-1 had started to spread, the CDC in the US said something worth remembering – 'We cannot keep bacteria from changing; bacteria will inevitably find ways of resisting the antibiotics developed by humans. This is why it is more important than ever to slow the spread of resistance by following infection control measures for every patient, every time, and to keep antibiotics working by improving how we use them.'

6

The Eye of the Storm

Shortly before the onset of the COVID-19 pandemic, a team of researchers at a US non-profit organization, the Center for Disease Dynamics, Economics and Policy, set out to assign a simple ranking of antibiotic resistance by country. Even though the problem of superbugs is a global one, there are disparities in healthcare and antibiotic use that have led to hotspots.

The researchers combined antibiotic consumption with resistance and assigned countries a number on a scale ranging from 0 to 100. The study was funded by the Bill and Melinda Gates Foundation and the CDC, and it was published in the *BMJ Global Health* journal. Sweden had the lowest resistance score of 8.1 while India had the highest at 71.6. A news story summarized the findings with the headline 'India tops the list of countries with highest antibiotic resistance, finds study'.

We can argue the merits of the approach that these researchers took and the relative position of India in a global ranking of resistance and superbugs. But one way or another, we must admit that India has a serious problem with superbugs.

Earlier, in 2017, the same organization provided an in-depth analysis of the superbug problem in India in a report titled 'Scoping Report on Antimicrobial Resistance in India'. This report was a part of a collaborative effort between India and the UK and highlighted the critical situation of antibacterial resistance in the country. It identified key areas where research was lacking. It included a foreword by K. VijayRaghavan, who was the secretary of the Department of Biotechnology at the Ministry of Science and Technology of the Government of India at the time. VijayRaghavan would later become the third Principal Scientific Adviser to the Government of India, a position he held during the COVID-19 pandemic.

The report was comprehensive, merging known information from multiple sources. It was designed to assist scientists and policymakers in India to develop targeted interventions against antibiotic resistance. The report acknowledged that while resistance in all kinds of microbes was concerning, the subset of bacterial resistance (which is the focus of this book) was the most serious health threat.

The report summarized the scale of the problem:

India has some of the highest antibiotic resistance rates among bacteria that commonly cause infections in the community and healthcare facilities. Resistance to the broad-spectrum antibiotics fluoroquinolones and third-generation cephalosporin was more than 70% in *Acinetobacter baumannii*, *Escherichia coli*, and *Klebsiella pneumoniae*, and more than 50% in *Pseudomonas aeruginosa*.

The report highlighted that the issue of superbugs had reached critical proportions and that resistance to carbapenems was also rising in Gram-negative bacteria, especially in four of the Deadly Six superbugs. The situation was further complicated by the emergence of resistance to colistin, the antibiotic used to treat infections when carbapenems didn't work (for example in superbugs that also contained NDM-1). The presence of colistin resistance led to bloodstream infections with *Klebsiella pneumoniae* with a staggering death rate of nearly 70 per cent among Indian patients. Fortunately, at the time, plasmid-mediated colistin resistance through MCR-1 or its variants was not prevalent in India. The report also found high levels of antibiotic-resistant superbugs in chickens and livestock. As we will discuss in Chapter 11, antibiotics are extensively used as growth promoters in agriculture.

Antibiotic-resistant superbugs were isolated from fish as well. Indian rivers, repositories of major biodiversity in the country, contained superbugs with high levels of resistance to critical antibiotics. Not only are antibiotic-resistant bacteria a concern, but the very genes that enable this resistance – including those resistant to last-resort antibiotics – were detected in major waterbodies, signalling an environmental crisis that accompanies the clinical challenge.

A considerable proportion of bacteria isolated from various water sources were antibiotic-resistant superbugs. Investigations across various Indian locales – from the historic stretches of Ayodhya and Faizabad to the bucolic landscapes of east Sikkim to the urban spread of Hyderabad – uncovered a disconcerting prevalence of antibiotic resistance among bacterial species like *E. coli* and *Klebsiella pneumoniae*. The report highlighted the intricate web connecting humans, animals, and the environment and the threat to health, mainly as a result of rampant antibiotic misuse. It should have been a wake-up call for the public but, unfortunately, it didn't leave a lasting impact.

India isn't only the world's most populous nation – Indians also have the highest rate of antibiotic consumption in the world with a median per capita consumption close to eleven units per year. (In this context, a 'unit' is the average daily dose of a drug as administered to adults, a standardized measure that allows for comparison of drug usage across different regions and times.) In fact, India single-handedly accounted for an astonishing 23 per cent of the global retail sales volume of antibiotics. And the numbers only keep growing.

The widespread use of these critical drugs is a product of a combination of factors. India is often referred to as the 'world's pharmacy' due to its massive drug manufacturing and distribution capacity. For a very long time, the country's pharmaceutical sales lacked stringent oversight. As a result, India makes a lot of antibiotics, and it's easy to get them without a prescription.

To understand how we've treated antibiotics in healthcare, I want to recount a folk story, supposedly about the seer Mullah Nasiruddin.

On a misty evening, with fog weaving through city streets, a young traveller trudged towards his home. The glow of a solitary street light was visible in the distance. As the traveller walked closer, he noticed that beneath that street light was a familiar figure, the quirky Mullah Nasiruddin.

'Mullah!' the traveller exclaimed, hurrying towards him. 'What on earth are you doing down there?'

Nasiruddin looked up, eyes filled with concern. 'I've misplaced my key,' he said with a sigh.

Seeing the Mullah's distress, the traveller crouched down beside him. For a while both quietly searched for the key under the glow of the street light. After what felt like an eternity, the traveller asked the sage a pertinent question. 'Mullah, it doesn't look like we are any closer to finding your key. Are you certain this is where you dropped it?'

Nasiruddin casually pointed towards the engulfing darkness and said, 'I dropped my key over there, inside my house.'

The traveller stared at him, dumbfounded. 'Inside your house? Then why are we searching out here?'

With an unmistakable twinkle in his eye, Mullah Nasiruddin replied, 'The light's far better out here, don't you think?'

This amusing story explains how we have come to treat antibiotics in India. We use them indiscriminately, not because they are always effective against the infections we suffer, but because they are easily available. Anyone familiar with the Indian landscape knows a major source of the problem. Antibiotics are sold over the counter at Indian pharmacies, with limited restrictions. Doctors prescribe them as a form of insurance often in low-resource settings.

One study estimated that just under half of the patients that walk into a doctor's office in Delhi get prescribed at least one antibiotic. As a result, patients are psychologically primed to expect antibiotics from doctors. Many medical professionals, often due to the insistence of their patients, resort to prescribing antibiotics even when they aren't necessary. People often believe that antibiotics are a cure-all solution and pressurize doctors to prescribe them based on prior experience or the incorrect notion that an infection that cleared up on its own was due to the effect of antibiotics.

Patients may come to expect antibiotics. Being prescribed medications is also seen as a sign of action as opposed to waiting to see if minor infections are self-limiting. Patients may also be reluctant to wait for diagnostic tests or they may lack the financial means to access them.

What's worse is that we often do this to ourselves, wilfully self-medicating with antibiotics at the first sign of illness. We all know how this process goes. After diarrhoea, or a cold, or a sore throat, many of us head off to the nearest pharmacy to 'self-prescribe' a course of antibiotics ourselves. And the neighbourhood pharmacy is happy to oblige the self-medication.

How do we know that the sore throat we have isn't the result of a viral infection or an allergy? We don't. The only way to be sure is to get a diagnosis based on a test. But do we test or culture for bacterial infections to rule out viruses at home? No, we don't. Despite the fact that the infection could've been caused by a virus, an allergy, or an irritant, we reach for the antibiotic because we can. No matter that it might be completely ineffective and worse, indiscriminate in killing off the bacteria that we harbour in our gut that are actually conducive to good health.

And it's not just any antibiotics. The 2017 report found that broad-spectrum antibiotics which should be used sparingly, were being used indiscriminately. These medicines, capable of targeting a wide variety of bacteria, had seen a spike in consumption, particularly with cephalosporins and broad-spectrum penicillins. In contrast, the use of narrow-spectrum penicillins, which are more targeted, had been low and on the decline.

Broad-spectrum antibiotics are vital when the specific bacterium causing an infection is unknown. However, they can accelerate the development of antibiotic resistance since their wide-reaching effect pushes many types of bacteria to evolve stronger defences. Additionally, they disturb friendly microbes, leading to secondary health issues, and potentially allowing resistant bacteria to thrive. This is discussed in greater detail in Chapter 8. Targeted, narrow-spectrum antibiotics, which are effective against specific bacteria, on the other hand, are generally more effective and less likely to contribute to resistance.

A significant portion of the antibiotics consumed in India are not even approved by central drug authorities. The 2017 report highlighted this as well, finding that the market was flooded with antibiotic fixed-dose combinations, which blend two or more antibiotics into a single dosage form. These should ideally be prescribed only when there is a clear benefit in effectiveness or safety over single antibiotics taken separately. Nevertheless, in India, these medicines are frequently prescribed without evidence of any such advantages, which likely makes the superbug problem worse.

The general lack of awareness about antibiotic misuse among the population, spanning urban and rural regions, also presents a huge challenge. For many, if not most Indians, the understanding of the limited role of antibiotics and the looming threat of superbugs is completely absent, or at best, very superficial. This haziness often translates to misuse and rampant overprescription. Street-side pharmacies, entirely lacking qualified medical practitioners, dispense antibiotics with abandon. Within the established confines of hospitals, an inadequate oversight of antibiotic administration exacerbates the issue.

The COVID-19 pandemic unleashed many medical and social challenges for the very first time. Therefore, it is not surprising that the interaction between the coronavirus and the use of antibiotics became prominent. Many patients were prescribed multiple antibiotics including azithromycin. But antibiotics don't work against viral diseases such as COVID-19. They can treat bacterial co-infections, but that was not a common occurrence during this pandemic (as it had been in past pandemics such as the Spanish flu pandemic of 1918–19).

This wasn't an isolated problem either – the prescription of antibiotics was shockingly widespread. There's research showing that around three out of every four COVID-19 patients globally were treated with antibiotics, regardless of whether they had another infection. I personally know of many people in India who were prescribed antibiotics during the second wave of COVID-19 in 2021 caused by the Delta variant of the virus.

Thus, it seems clear that there isn't a single root cause for the misuse of antibiotics. The rampant and unnecessary use of these drugs stems from a combination of poor medical practices, gaps in public awareness, and systemic challenges in sanitation. Addressing these issues requires multifaceted interventions, ranging from educating the public to improving hygiene standards in healthcare facilities.

The Indian Council of Medical Research (ICMR), through its Antimicrobial Resistance Research and Surveillance Network, is deeply involved in understanding how certain bacteria in India are becoming resistant to antibiotics. At the time of writing this book, the ICMR's latest report had focused on infections in larger hospitals during 2022. The ICMR found that the Deadly Six bacteria were increasingly resistant to drugs. This report, while specific to large hospitals, reveals trends that could affect the broader healthcare landscape in India.

Of over one lakh bacterial samples studied, resistant *E. coli* was the most common culprit, but there was also a significant presence of other dangerous bacteria. The report reveals a concerning trend. *E. coli* and *Klebsiella pneumoniae* are becoming increasingly resistant to imipenem, which is a type of carbapenem antibiotic.

This resistance has grown over the last five years. In 2017, about 81 per cent of *E. coli* bacteria could be fought with imipenem, but by 2022, that number had fallen to 66 per cent. The situation is similar for *Klebsiella pneumoniae*, where resistance has increased even more, with the drug only effective against 42 per cent of these bacteria in 2022, down from 59 per cent in 2017. The report also details how some bacteria, particularly *Pseudomonas aeruginosa* and *Acinetobacter baumannii*, were becoming superbugs, with the latter showing around 88 per cent resistance rate to carbapenems. This suggests limited options for treating infections caused by these bacteria, especially in ICUs.

The report didn't just highlight problems, however. It also pointed out some limited successes. Levonadifloxacin is an antibiotic developed in India that took over a decade to come to market. Approved in 2019, it's now aiding physicians in treating MRSA. The latest ICMR report showed that relatively new antibiotics like levonadifloxacin were showing promise in fighting this deadly superbug.

India grapples with a significant burden of infections, which can largely be attributed to various issues including poor hygiene standards, subpar sanitation facilities, and rampant overcrowding. Such conditions form a breeding ground for infections, thereby elevating the demand for antibiotics. Due to concerns about cleanliness and the potential risk of infections in many medical facilities, healthcare professionals tend to prescribe antibiotics as a precautionary measure.

On digging deeper, it is clear that issues in the Indian health system are just the initial and most visible layer of a more profound problem. The exponential increase in antibiotic use in India is not just a tale of inadequate regulations. Over the years, the country has witnessed an impressive growth in income levels. The nation's economy has been on an upward trajectory, and this economic growth has given its citizens more purchasing power. However, many experts believe that this rise in income has not been met with corresponding investments in public health.

Compared with other similar-sized economies, particularly in the BRICS categorization (Brazil, Russia,

India, China, and South Africa), India's performance in fundamental health metrics appears to be lagging. The country trails behind its counterparts on essential health indicators, such as sanitation facilities and immunization coverage. These are foundational elements for a healthy populace, and neglect in these areas invariably leads to a higher predisposition to infections.

India's complex healthcare ecosystem, marked by diverse systems, governance transitions, and big regional disparities in access to healthcare often impedes the uniform adoption of policy reforms. Additionally, telling doctors to limit antibiotic prescriptions without equipping them with rapid diagnostic tools presents a challenge for these professionals as well.

However, simple actions do have an impact as well, and this is especially true when it comes to prevention. Awareness campaigns championing hand hygiene can build on the experiences of the COVID-19 pandemic. The challenge of access to clean water and sanitation is also being addressed. In this respect, the Swachh Bharat Mission was a much-needed step in the right direction.

Given increasing mobile phone access, technology could also play a greater role in monitoring antibiotic use and surveillance of superbugs. Mobile phone use is widespread these days and mobiles can be used by healthcare professionals to report antibiotic use and occurrences of outbreaks. Mobile apps were used to great effect for contact tracing during the COVID-19 pandemic and digitization of vaccine records.

On the regulatory front, efforts to streamline antibiotic use have also been initiated. Prohibitions on specific high-risk drug combinations and stricter controls on antibiotic sales have been put in place. Schedule H1, for instance, is a regulatory measure that curtails over-the-counter antibiotic sales. While some states like Kerala have strictly implemented these regulations, enforcement, primarily due to resource constraints, remains lax in other regions.

Resource allocation, in fact, remains a significant challenge. Initiatives for infectious disease awareness and surveillance and government-sponsored biomedical research must compete for funding with other critical needs such as education, employment, and infrastructure. Battling superbugs hasn't emerged as a top-tier priority for many governments. In the absences of budgets earmarked for combating antibiotic resistance, progress has been slow.

The COVID-19 pandemic only exacerbated this, diverting attention and resources, relegating the challenge of antibiotic resistance into the shadows. India's strategy in dealing with antibiotic resistance involved including antimicrobial stewardship programmess within hospitals. These programmes focus on equipping hospital staff with the knowledge of judicious antibiotic use, emphasizing the need for resistance testing for bacteria, following prescribing guidelines, and monitoring of antibiotic use. These initiatives were deprioritized to focus on the COVID-19 pandemic.

Just when the world should've focused more on stopping superbugs, we shifted our attention and the problem started to get worse.

7

The World Outside

Antibiotics are drugs, but to the microbes that make them, they're a vital resource. To understand how to properly use antibiotics, we need to know how and why they're made in the natural world. This kind of appreciation, unfortunately, is woefully lacking in most populations. So, why *do* some microbes make antibiotics?

Antibiotics are what biologists call 'secondary metabolites', meaning they are not necessary for the immediate survival of the organisms that produce them. For the longest time, the answer to why some microbes are so good at making antibiotics seemed simple. Scientists believed that antibiotics gave the microbes that made them an edge in the battle for precious resources by wiping out the competition.

We are used to extracting resources from our environment and packaging them in ways that bear little resemblance to their original states. So, we might not ask this question in our daily lives, but it's a useful way to appreciate the natural world. For example, some plants make caffeine, which gives us a high, and chilli peppers produce capsaicin, the chemical that gives them their unmistakable kick. But what's the point of these products from the plants' perspective?

This is one of the big questions that biologists often ask. Here's a maxim in biology: if an organism makes something that requires energy, it is likely either helpful in some way or it's an evolutionary leftover from a time when it was useful.

Life is a struggle. Whether you're a plant, animal, or a tiny single-celled microbe, you're always up against a harsh environment, and there are other living things competing for the same resources. So why would any organism spend precious energy making something that isn't essential for its immediate survival?

Invisible to the naked eye, a gram of soil can contain up to 10 billion microbes belonging to thousands of different species, putting the diversity of the visible world to shame. These microbes include not only bacteria, but also fungi, protozoa, algae, and nematodes. And for every bacterium in the environment, there are at least ten viruses, making them the most prevalent biological entities on the planet.

How would one kind of bacteria be expected to survive in this crowded environment filled with many hostile entities? 'By making large amounts of weapons' might be the first answer that you could expect from humans. When we first discovered antibiotics, they seemed like magic bullets that could wipe out harmful bacteria with incredible efficiency. Consequently, when we used them, to us it was like deploying a nuclear bomb against microscopic foes.

It would help if we knew exactly which microbes we were dealing with when we examined the natural world. But we're only accustomed to looking at a small slice of life at this microscopic scale. Traditionally, microbiologists would try to grow bacteria by providing specific conditions and food in the lab that they could use to grow. This process helped scientists select individual strains of bacteria, which, in turn, helped tease apart their stories. In fact, this is the bedrock of the techniques used in microbiology.

In the process of selecting specific strains, however, biologists were excluding perhaps 99 per cent of the microbes that existed in natural environments. Scientists also soon figured out that they could not easily replicate the complex interactions between microbes in the natural world within their pristine lab settings.

The middle of the last century was the 'golden age' of antibiotics, a time when new antibiotics were being discovered constantly. And just when it seemed like there was going to be a limitless supply of new antibiotics only waiting to be unearthed, the discoveries slowed down. When searching for new antibiotics, scientists often ended up isolating and identifying known drugs. This was because many of the easier-to-find antibiotics had already been identified. The undiscovered antibiotics were either more elusive, or they existed in environments that were harder to access. So, within a few years, it became harder to find new antibiotics that had never been seen before. It seemed then as if we had found every natural antibiotic that was easily available to us.

It would be fine if the ones we had discovered kept working as well as they did when we found them. Then we would not need to discover new antibiotics. But as we are finding out that turned out not to be the case. In Lewis Carroll's *Through the Looking-Glass*, the Red Queen tells Alice, 'Now, here, you see, it takes all the running you can do, to keep in the same place.' This notion became emblematic of what scientists later termed the 'Red Queen Effect', a phenomenon in which organisms must constantly adapt and evolve just to maintain the status quo in relation to their co-evolving competitors or adversaries.

The search for new antibiotics is driven by the Red Queen Effect. Bacteria have been on Earth for billions of years and have evolved sophisticated mechanisms to survive. As a result, even as scientists develop and introduce new antibiotics, bacterial populations work to swiftly counteract them. Thus, much like Alice found herself running but not making any progress, scientists often find they remain in a seemingly perpetual battle against ever-resilient bacterial foes despite their efforts in developing new drugs.

To understand the urgency of this problem, one need only pay attention to the rise of superbugs, which as we've

The World Outside

discussed, resist the effects of multiple antibiotics. The rapid evolution of these organisms means that even as we create new treatments, the goalposts are continually shifting.

However, the question still remains: if antibiotics are a precious resource created by microbes, where did the resistance genes that serve as antidotes come from? The answer is also microbes.

You might think that resistance genes magically appeared as soon as we started using antibiotics. But the truth is more complex. Many of these defences have been part of bacterial DNA for a long, long time, indeed for longer than humans have been in existence. Bacteria have a remarkable skill for creating antibiotics. They also have a remarkable talent for adapting, evolving, and sharing genetic tools to defend themselves against antibiotics. The deep-rooted history and intricate ways in which bacteria manoeuvre to resist drugs provide insights into the dynamic world of invisible life forms.

Antibiotics were made and used long before we discovered them. Erythromycin, streptomycin, and vancomycin, for example, are ancient, with their origins dating back hundreds of millions of years. As these antibiotic-producing bacteria emerged, they often had to counteract the poisons they were producing themselves. Other bacteria had to find ways to survive too. This led to the early development of resistance tools, some of which date back over 2 billion years.

A compelling theory suggests that bacteria-producing

antibiotics might be the origin of many resistance genes, and it makes sense if we think about it. If a bacterium is producing a toxic substance like an antibiotic, it needs a mechanism to protect itself. Over time, these defensive tools would be shared with other bacteria, allowing them to withstand the toxic effects of antibiotics.

Given the ancient nature of antibiotics and the rapid replication ability of bacteria, it's not surprising that resistance has become so widespread. Biology is thrifty. Just as the genetic blueprints that give rise to antibiotics were likely repurposed from genetic blueprints with other roles, it is also quite possible that the genes that give rise to antibiotic resistance were modified from other genes. In other words, resistance likely evolved from other biological tools that originally had different jobs, gradually transforming into the sophisticated resistance systems we see today.

Resistance is shared, and there are multiple pathways to sharing these traits. There are several layers to these processes, some of which are like nested dolls that fit one inside another. As we discussed in Chapter 2, resistance genes can be a part of hopping elements called transposons. These can be a part of various plasmids that get swapped between bacteria. These mobile elements can be nested within one another and even picked up from other bacteria in intermediate hosts. And of course, bacteria can also share genes with their offspring.

Here's the crux of the matter. Contrary to popular opinion, most bacteria don't just mutate to become resistant. They pick up their resistance genes from other bacteria. These genetic materials come from nature itself and can even be found in isolated places like caves. This striking fact has been accentuated by many studies including a recent one on the emergence of one of our Deadly Six superbugs, methicillin-resistant *Staphylococcus aureus* or MRSA.

For a brief time, methicillin, an antibiotic closely related to penicillin, was the go-to solution to combat certain bacteria like *Staphylococcus aureus*. But it didn't take long before the resistance to methicillin became widespread. Enter MRSA, a superbug that has stumped medical professionals for years.

Where did MRSA come from? Although it's tempting to blame the birth of MRSA solely on the modern use of antibiotics, this would be far from the truth. A landmark study traced this superbug's lineage far beyond hospitals and farms where antibiotics are routinely used. In 2022, an international consortium of researchers from the University of Cambridge, the Wellcome Sanger Institute, Denmark's Statens Serum Institut, the University of Oxford, and the Royal Botanic Gardens at Kew made a startling discovery. MRSA pre-dates the use of antibiotics by at least one hundred years!

The culprit? Those incredibly cute and perilously cuddly hedgehogs. Surveys conducted in Denmark and Sweden showed that up to 60 per cent of these creatures carry a strain of MRSA. And the plot thickens. High levels of MRSA were also detected in hedgehog populations across Europe and even in New Zealand.

There are certain facts we need to consider in order to see this story in context. Contrary to popular wisdom, not all bacteria are harmful or deadly. While hand sanitizer commercials might depict bacteria as menacing, cartoonish threats that must be quashed with 99.9 per cent effectiveness, the truth is most bacteria don't cause disease in humans. In fact, many simply coexist with us. For example, *Staphylococcus aureus* can live on the skin of humans and hedgehogs without causing any harm. But in certain circumstances, strains of this bacteria can resourcefully become the cause of disease. Nature does indeed abhor a vacuum.

So, what turns *Staphylococcus aureus* into the dreaded superbug MRSA on hedgehogs? What the researchers hypothesized as the spark that led to the superbug is a battle that takes place on the skin of hedgehogs. There, along with *Staphylococcus aureus* is a fungus known as *Trichophyton erinaceid*, which produces its own antibiotics. To survive in this environment, the bacteria had to evolve resistance or perish. As Ewan Harrison, a senior author of the study, put it, 'It wasn't the use of penicillin that drove the initial emergence of MRSA; it was a natural biological process.'

The takeaway here is sobering yet crucial. Antibiotic resistance is both natural and inevitable. We should remember that some form of resistance to all antibiotics we can hope to isolate from natural sources already probably exists. We cannot unwind the clock to reverse hundreds of millions of years of evolution or change the rules of coexistence of life on the planet. If antibiotics exist, then antibiotic resistance also exists. What we *can* control, however, is how we use antibiotics, a pivotal factor in preventing the spread of antibiotic resistance and the resulting rapid proliferation of superbugs that render vital treatments ineffective.

Scientists think that natural antibiotics were made by microbes for many millions of years. Yet, in just a few years of humans discovering and using them as medicines, bacterial resistance has skyrocketed, greatly limiting their effectiveness. In addition, the swift emergence of multidrug resistance in superbugs can be directly tied to human use. But the patterns of use that have been repeated after every single antibiotic is discovered also lead us to believe that resistance is inevitable.

So why did we still find antibiotics like penicillin effective when we discovered them nearly a century ago? Why haven't more bacteria in nature become entirely resistant to these antibiotics over millions of years like so many superbugs have after only a few years of human use? Do bacteria in nature manage antibiotics in a way that somehow maintains their effectiveness? Why hasn't resistance spread to the point where natural antibiotics are useless?

These questions are important since they help us understand how antibiotics function in both natural ecosystems and human environments. They show how we might perhaps be able to preserve the effectiveness of antibiotics for as long as possible.

Evolution hinges on variation, and in bacteria, this

variation comes from two primary sources. The first is mutations, which can happen quickly due to bacteria's short generation times, enabling the rapid development of new protective traits. For example, a single mutation can change the way a bacterium interacts with an antibiotic, rendering the drug ineffective.

But the most frightening way that variations occur in bacteria is via the sharing of mobile genetic elements. A population always has variations. Let's assume that a resistance gene exists in some bacteria in a population but not in others. Threats like industrial-grade antibiotics act as selective pressures, endowing the bacteria with effective defence mechanisms. Those that don't have these mechanisms fail to thrive.

Evolution does not offer a straightforward path to the ultimate defence system. Defensive traits often come with trade-offs. For example, a bacterium that evolves to resist one type of antibiotic might become more susceptible to another. On the flip side, a single defence mechanism might offer protection against multiple threats.

Antibiotic resistance exists naturally, but human action tips the scales from it being a sporadic event to a hidden pandemic of superbugs. For bacteria, maintaining resistance genes requires energy and resources. In the long run, resistance is an insurance policy that only pays off if antibiotics are present in large quantity. And since antibiotics have been used commercially, it has become a good insurance policy for bacteria to have resistance.

The antibiotic era began with the discovery of penicillin by Alexander Fleming in 1928. While being initially challenging to produce and purify, the collaborative efforts of several chemists eventually made penicillin widely available. Its effectiveness was mostly against Gram-positive bacteria, and it took a few more years for researchers to discover antibiotics such as streptomycin, which are effective against Gram-negative bacteria.

However, our resistance to antibiotics became apparent almost immediately after we started using them. At first, it didn't matter that much because we were discovering new antibiotics at a fast pace. Unfortunately, this well of new antibiotics dried up by the 1970s, and since then, very few new antibiotics have been found.

Public health officials have tried to control antibiotic use in hopes of reducing resistance, but this strategy hasn't worked as expected. The logic was that if we used fewer antibiotics, the bacteria would revert to being non-resistant. However, that's not what happens. It appears that once bacteria evolve to be resistant, they don't easily go back to being susceptible to antibiotics even when the antibiotics are removed from their environment.

We have now started to appreciate that defensive traits like antibiotic resistance tend to stick around even when they're no longer needed. In essence, once bacteria gain a specific kind of resistance, getting rid of it is not easy. The best way to deal with resistance is to prevent its spread for as long as possible.

A general theme of this book is that microbes are better at making complex molecules like antibiotics than we are. But if we believe that resistance is a counterbalance to antibiotics that emerges naturally, you can see that there's a big problem. The same diversity in environments that ensures that we will find new antibiotics ensures that there are already some bacteria that are resistant to them.

So, the next time you read a headline in a news story announcing a new antibiotic for which there are no known resistant bacteria, mentally add in the word 'yet'. Resistance to natural antibiotics lurks in the wild, and there's only a narrow window of time for use in medicine before the genes that impart resistance are spread widely.

One thing is clear: if we know antibiotic resistance is coming and once it is widespread it is hard to reverse, we should hear the clock ticking for every effective antibiotic. The only way to stretch out the time period of effectiveness of antibiotics is to ensure we use them in a way that resistance doesn't spread rapidly. And for this, we can look to nature.

In the wild, the usage of antibiotics greatly differs from how they are applied in medical scenarios. To point out a stark contrast, antibiotics in nature are not generated in massive amounts, nor do they last indefinitely. In healthcare, antibiotics are administered primarily to eradicate all susceptible bacteria with all other effects being secondary. Recognizing this difference between nature and the clinic can shed light on the potential variations in outcomes.

When it comes to medical treatment, antibiotics are given in high doses over a fixed time period, which is determined historically. There is also a significant focus on the interplay between the concentration of the antibiotic and its duration. The optimal dosage for effectively combating an infection revolves around the antibiotic's potency in eradicating bacteria and its strength within the body.

So, it is essential for the concentration of an antibiotic to consistently be above a minimum inhibitory concentration to thwart a disease-causing bacterium within a patient. To get to where the antibiotic needs to be to fight infection, the antibiotic concentration is kept at a high level through the course of treatment and the concentration tapers in time after each dose until the next dose enters the body.

However, the concentration of antibiotics in nature is believed to be much lower than in clinical settings where the dosage must surpass a threshold concentration to stop an infection. Such high concentrations of antibiotics are rare in nature, typically found only very close to the microbe producing them.

In nature, there's a gradient of antibiotic concentration spread out over the area. Concentrations are high close to the bacteria that produce the antibiotic, but they drop further away. Within patients, antibiotics are meant to be distributed throughout the body to kill bacteria where they find them. This is key to understanding bacterial survival and why they are pressured to evolve and acquire resistance when people use antibiotics.

While human and animal systems break down and excrete antibiotics, natural settings, like the soil around us, provide a more prolonged but less concentrated antibiotic presence. Some antibiotics break down slowly in soil and can last for many years. Environmental factors like temperature, moisture, and pH impact the speed at which antibiotics degrade, making it a slow and inconsistent process.

We can see how our use of these drugs has driven the spread of antibiotic resistance and the rise of superbugs. In nature, a bacterium lacking resistance to an antibiotic present in low concentrations might not die as a result. In contrast, for disease-causing bacteria in the human body, lacking resistance means the bacteria will perish.

And this is not limited to the antibiotics we consume. Our environment is awash with antibiotics. The widespread industrial use of antibiotics in livestock farming especially has consistently introduced them into natural ecosystems at unnatural concentrations, upsetting the balance of naturally produced antibiotics and their resistance mechanisms. Due to its lasting consequences, this mismanagement has been compared to nuclear weapons testing. Just as nuclear weapons testing leaves behind radiation that can affect the environment and human health for decades, polluting the environment with excessive antibiotics can have repercussions that last into the future. Since large-scale antibiotic production began in 1942, exposure to these drugs has left an indelible mark on life.

Long-term data reveals that natural antibiotic production often occurs in tandem with a matching resistance mechanism. Over time, the balance between antibiotic production and the development of resistance likely stayed stable because the forces driving change were even. Significant changes in either direction would be costly in terms of energy and resources to the microbes and would not be beneficial. In nature, there is likely an equilibrium between antibiotic production and resistance.

However, human intervention disrupted this ancient microbial 'social contract'. We appropriated antibiotics, assuming them to be underutilized, and turned them into potent agents that encouraged bacteria to develop resistance. This set in motion an unavoidable spiral of escalating resistance levels.

Many scientists now believe that some antibiotics may be used by microbes to communicate and work together. Some antibiotics also pass messages between microbes and larger organisms like plants and insects. So, while we once thought of antibiotics simply as microbial weapons of mass destruction, we're beginning to understand that they have a more nuanced role in the microscopic world – somewhere between a weapon, a messenger and a mystery yet to be solved.

Interestingly, the actinomycetes – the specialized category of bacteria that make more antibiotics than any other group – seem to have first appeared around the time when plants first moved on to land, which is around 440 million years ago.

Many of these bacteria bind themselves to plant roots, and it would make sense that some of the compounds they make would be used to communicate with plants.

Thus, for example, consider how antibiotics spread through soil. Bacteria release the antibiotic, which spreads out from the source. This creates a zone around the bacteria where other microbes struggle to survive. But as we move further from the source, the antibiotic keeps spreading at lower concentrations, affecting even those microbes that are farther away. In medicine, we try to maintain a constant high dose of the antibiotic within the body.

In the natural world, being closely related, or having a history of cooperation could make microbes more likely to live together. Antibiotics could serve as a sort of police force that regulates zoning. You could see it as microbial communities using antibiotics to decide who to let in and who to keep out.

The task of finding new antibiotics is getting harder, forcing scientists to look in new places. First, scientists are starting to explore new potential sources of antibiotics that have not been studied before. Most antibiotics come from a few bacterial species in soil. But most of the world's soils have not been screened for microbes that have the potential to make antibiotics.

Casting the net wider could help us to find new bacterial strains and new types of antibiotics. Besides soils, ocean environments have shown promise. For instance, compounds have been isolated from certain ocean-dwelling bacteria that are now being tested for their anti-microbial and anti-cancer potential. Similarly, the bacteria that live as beneficial partners with sea creatures, or even within our own bodies, could be a rich source of new natural compounds. Many bacteria also live close to plants and small animals such as insects, and these are also currently being tested.

Studying microbes that we can't grow in the lab can be done by examining the genetic material found in environmental samples, like soil or water. This method has become feasible thanks to advancements in DNA analysis technology. We can think of DNA as a set of instructions to guide the construction of useful biological molecules. These instructions can tell us a lot about how an organism functions, including how it might produce antibiotics.

With modern technology, scientists have become adept at rapidly sequencing the DNA of microbes known to produce antibiotics. So, they can search for DNA instructions with the potential to produce new antibiotics. These instructions are then compared with those of known antibiotics. If scientists find DNA sequences similar to those of known antibiotics, it suggests that these instructions from microbes might encode similar antibiotic compounds, even if we can't grow the microbes that they belong to in a laboratory. This method opens up a whole new world of discovering potential antibiotics directly from nature.

It turns out many bacteria have a wealth of untapped

genetic instructions that could potentially produce a variety of natural compounds including antibiotics. While we've identified many of the instructions for creating enzymes that look like they could be useful in making antibiotics, the pieces don't often fit.

These puzzling instructions could be for 'hidden antibiotics' that we haven't yet coaxed microbes into making. This often seems as if the microbes have secret instructions that we can't fully understand yet. Awakening these 'sleeping' genes has become an exciting area of research, holding out the hope of discovering new drugs.

In addition, scientists are speeding up the pace of mining for new antibiotics using advanced DNA analysis techniques that try to unearth hidden antibiotics. Most bacteria that exist in nature are hard to grow in the lab. Some of these bacteria have shown the genetic potential to produce new kinds of antibiotics when coaxed under the right conditions.

Extracting DNA directly from environmental samples like soil, analysing this DNA to find genes that might produce new antibiotics, and then using other bacteria in the lab to produce these substances helped scientists discover a new class of antibiotics called malacidins. This discovery is exciting because it shows there's a huge potential to find new antibiotics from nature that we haven't been able to access before.

Overall, we need to rethink our approach to these drugs. Instead of viewing antibiotics only as weapons against harmful bacteria, we should consider their broader role in shaping microbial communities and entire environments. The key point to remember, though, is that while antibiotic resistance is normal and precedes human use of antibiotics, our use has certainly accelerated the process.

8

The World Within Us

Each person is a vast ecosystem that hosts trillions of different kinds of microbes – bacteria, viruses, and fungi – that live in our gut, skin, and other parts of the body. These microscopic residents, collectively known as the microbiome, generally live in harmony with us. In addition, these microbes provide several health benefits that have become more apparent to scientists over the past few decades. Connections between our microbes, especially those in our gut, and many aspects of our health are being discovered with astonishing frequency. This is one of the most exciting areas of science today and a space in medicine to watch in the future.

The composition of microbes in the microbiome and how microbiomes change over time and during disease and ageing is a subject of intense discussion today. Rarely does a month go by without a landmark study being published in a leading science journal highlighting a new facet of the inextricable link between the microbes inside us and our health. Very broadly speaking, there's a balance maintained in the population of microbes within the body of a healthy person.

By now, you might assume that the improper and frequent use of antibiotics only harms environments and groups of people. You might be under the assumption that by popping those pills you're not immediately harming your own health. While it's true that antibiotics are essential in treating many bacterial infections that wouldn't get better on their own, antibiotics can also cause a wide-ranging set of problems by disrupting the balance of the microbes that call our bodies home.

Most courses of antibiotics will not result in the person taking them getting so sick that additional problems arise. Before convincing yourself that taking a few antibiotics you found at home is harmless when dealing with a sore throat or unexplained diarrhoea, it's crucial to recognize the personal risks involved. You see, antibiotics don't discriminate between disease-causing bacteria and beneficial ones. Even as they defeat the bacterial infection for which they're being taken, they also target friendly microbes, upsetting the delicate balance of the microbiome. This disruption can sometimes lead to other health problems. For instance, changes in our gut microbiomes have been linked to conditions like obesity, diabetes, and asthma.

That's not the only issue you need to look out for. When antibiotics disrupt the balance of the microbiome, they heighten the risk of catching other infections. Antibiotics can suppress the good bacteria that keep other harmful microbes in check, and can increase the risk of other bacterial, fungal, and even viral infections.

When you take antibiotics, you're applying the pressure of evolutionary selection that favours bacteria resistant to the drugs. Over time, as more and more bacteria are exposed to antibiotics, the chances of some acquiring resistance genes and becoming superbugs is greater. This is an issue for communities, countries, and the entire world for sure. But it's also something to come to terms with personally.

Antibiotics are essential to modern medicine, but we need to understand the collateral damage caused every time we take them. Even one round of antibiotics can boost the growth of resistant superbugs that are already in someone's body. This is not just a global health problem but a direct, immediate risk to the patient.

Further, with the rampant use of antibiotics, there's now a significant chance that individuals might already have superbugs in their bodies before starting treatment. These superbugs can cause hard-to-treat infections, especially during or shortly after antibiotic treatment. The result might be a superinfection that is even harder to treat than the initial illness.

The impact antibiotics have on our microbiomes depends

on a few factors. For instance, how and where the antibiotic enters the body, how the body processes it and gets rid of it, and its range of activity can all influence the outcome of our microbiomes and our health. Some antibiotics come in the form of pills or capsules that are directly introduced into the digestive system after they're swallowed. If they're not fully absorbed, there may be a high concentration of the antibiotic in the gut which can linger and harm friendly bacteria colonizing the gut. Other antibiotics, administered via injection, might only indirectly affect gut bacteria based on how they're processed and eliminated from the body.

The way our bodies respond to antibiotics varies considerably from one person to another. Take the antibiotic ceftriaxone, for instance. Ceftriaxone is an antibiotic of the cephalosporin class that is used to treat a wide range of bacterial infections. When you take ceftriaxone, it is absorbed into the bloodstream and distributed throughout the body. The liver then breaks down the drug, and one of the pathways for elimination is that it is excreted into bile. A digestive fluid produced by the liver, bile is released into the intestines where it aids in digestion. The presence of ceftriaxone in the bile results from the liver's role in drug metabolism and excretion. The amount of the drug excreted in the bile can vary significantly in people due to differences in liver function, genetic factors, and other individual health variables influencing how the drug affects the gut microbiota. Antibiotics in the bile can alter the bacterial environment in the gut since they can affect both harmful bacteria (their intended target) and beneficial bacteria (an unintended side effect).

Plus, each person's microbiome is unique. Research suggests that the specific types of species in our microbiomes and how they interact with each other plays a part in how stable our microbial environment is and how microbes react to disturbances like antibiotics. Studies have shown that when a group of healthy volunteers were given the same antibiotic, their gut microbiomes responded differently. In some cases, a few volunteers experienced strong changes and their pretreatment microbial diversity took a long time to recover.

We know that certain people might face more significant adverse effects from antibiotics than others. Infants and older adults, for example, often show less stability in their microbiomes as compared to healthy younger adults. Another twist in the tale is the presence of antibiotic-resistant bacteria within the host microbiome. While these bacteria can lead to hard-to-treat infections, they also affect how antibiotics impact the gut. Resistant bacteria can share their resistance traits with harmful bacteria, turning them into superbugs. However, at the same time, if an antibiotic doesn't affect these resistant bacteria, it means they can keep doing their job, maintaining a balance in our microbial community. Some bacteria even help their neighbours by producing enzymes that break down antibiotics, effectively shielding the community from the effects of the drug.

Several factors shape the composition of our microbiomes. For example, if we're around livestock on a farm or in areas with contaminated sewage, we might pick up not only new types of microbes but also their antibiotic resistance genes. Since the microbiome's starting point determines how antibiotics affect it, these environmental factors influence our personal antibiotic experience as well.

Interestingly, a specific side effect of antibiotic usage can provide some insight into its impact on microbiomes. A common side effect of antibiotics is diarrhoea, occurring, by some estimates, in around a third of people who take antibiotics and caused by the disruption to the gut microbiome from antibiotic use. Taking multiple, different antibiotics at once only increases the chances of experiencing this side effect. This issue is worsened with the use of fixed-dose combinations of two or more antibiotics, most of which are widely available in India.

Another factor in the disruption to the body is the range or spectrum of activity of the antibiotic. Our intestines house a majority of bacteria that are anaerobes, meaning they thrive in environments that lack oxygen like the gut. Some antibiotics broadly target these anaerobes, including the essential ones we need, which can lead to an increase in other bacteria – harmful ones that can tolerate oxygen.

There is a relationship between our microbiomes and our immune system as well. The two influence each other in multiple ways. Our immune system helps regulate our microbiome, ensuring it remains balanced. In return, microbes play a role in shaping our immune responses. So, an individual's immune status, or any other health conditions, can influence how their microbiome reacts to antibiotics. For example, the gut microbiome of someone undergoing chemotherapy might differ significantly from a healthy individual, changing the way they respond to antibiotic treatment.

The effect of antibiotics can also be influenced by other medications. Some drugs, like anti-inflammatory drugs or antipsychotics, can affect specific bacteria in our gut. Combining these drugs with antibiotics can alter their combined impact on our system. A common example is proton pump inhibitors which reduce stomach acid production. These drugs, commonly sold as antacids, when taken with antibiotics, can amplify certain side effects, like antibiotic-associated diarrhoea. However, these combined effects are often not mentioned by prescribing doctors.

While antibiotics are essential protection from harmful bacteria, they can also provoke other bacteria in our bodies into turning into potential threats. Many bacteria that can cause diseases are often found living harmlessly inside us. The majority of the deaths caused by bacteria worldwide can be traced back to just a few strains of bacteria that usually reside peacefully in healthy people. In many cases, the infections caused by these bacteria aren't picked up from somewhere else; instead, they arise from the very same bacterial populations that have been living inside us until that point without causing any issues.

Let's take *Staphylococcus aureus*, which can become MRSA, one of our Deadly Six superbugs. A study observed some patients known to carry the bacteria in their noses. Among those who later developed a bloodstream infection with this bacterium, a staggering 83 per cent had strains in their blood matching the ones in their noses, sometimes even more than a year earlier. Similarly, a type of *E. coli* responsible for urinary tract infections is often found quietly living in the gut. The infections had not come from elsewhere – they had come from bacteria living within that had transformed into superbugs.

In another study, a patient suffering from recurring urinary infections had an *E. coli* strain that moved between their gut and bladder for a staggering five years! In the gut, the bacterium was harmless, but in the bladder, it caused a serious infection.

Now, the big question is: what triggers these usually peaceful bacteria to suddenly turn problematic? There are some clues that reveal the answer for this behaviour.

Various factors within our body can push potential bacterial troublemakers to change their behaviour from being simple, harmless tenants to ones causing severe infections. We know that the acquisition of resistance genes causes bacteria to become superbugs. Having a healthy mix of bacteria living inside our bodies plays a protective role, shielding us from many invasive harmful bacteria. This protective shield created by our body's native bacteria is something scientists call 'colonization resistance'. Here's a colourful way to think about this. Imagine your gut as a vast beach with trillions of tiny beach chairs in which friendly bacteria relax and luxuriate. When these friendly bacteria are wiped out, those chairs remain, ready for other harmful microbes to occupy them.

When a balance of good bacteria is maintained, they defend us in a couple of ways. First, they can directly challenge the harmful ones by competing for the same nutrients, or by producing substances that act like natural antibiotics. Second, they indirectly bolster our body's defences, prepping our immune system to fight off infections.

Unfortunately, antibiotic usage sometimes harms the good bacteria, disrupting this colonization resistance. When this balance is upset, we become much more vulnerable to infections. Studies from as far back as the 1950s have shown that animals treated with antibiotics were more susceptible to infections by certain harmful bacteria compared to those which had not been treated.

A classic example of this phenomenon in humans is the infection caused by the bacteria *Clostridioides difficile* (also known as *C. diff*). After taking certain antibiotics, some people become highly prone to this infection, which can lead to severe digestive issues. There are estimates that between 10 per cent and 25 per cent of all cases of antibiotic-associated diarrhoea are due to an underlying *Clostridioides difficile* infection that flared up after infections, leading to a painful condition called colitis.

In addition, certain antibiotics like clindamycin are especially notorious for creating the right atmosphere for these later infections. And the severity and duration of the antibiotic treatment further increases the risk. Interestingly, one of the remedies for such infections is to reintroduce a mix of healthy bacteria into the affected individuals. This can be done either by giving them a concoction of specific bacteria or, in more extreme cases, using faecal transplants from healthy donors.

Clostridioides difficile isn't the only harmful bacterium that can attack when our good bacteria are down. Other bacteria like *Klebsiella* and MRSA could also be behind some cases of digestive issues following antibiotic use. Animal studies have shown that antibiotics can pave the way for *Salmonella* infections as well.

It is bad enough when the problem occurs in one part of the body, and it is self-limiting like a case of diarrhoea. But sometimes, the issue isn't just localized. Disease-causing bacteria that have multiplied in one part of the body can travel to other parts too. For example, some bacteria are harmless where they usually live in the gut. However, when they grow due to antibiotic use, they can enter the bloodstream, leading to serious infections. This jump from the gut to the bloodstream can be caused by a weakened gut barrier after the bacteria's normal environment is disrupted by antibiotics.

Similarly, bacteria can move from the gut to other areas like the urinary or respiratory tracts. For example, when harmful bacteria multiply in the gut, they get expelled in our waste. This could increase the chances of these bacteria reaching and infecting other parts of our body like the urinary system. It is important to note that our urinary system isn't sterile. It benefits from colonization resistance too. Notably, women who've been treated with antibiotics for other ailments are more likely to develop urinary tract infections afterwards, with some studies indicating a three- to sixfold increased risk. Additionally, in places like hospitals, this high shedding of bacteria due to antibiotic use can also increase the risk of infections spreading to other patients.

So far, we've talked mostly about the gut, but the skin, our body's largest organ, isn't simply a passive barrier. It hosts a community of microbes that actively defend us against pathogens. Many of these resident microbes process proteins and lipids found on our skin to produce substances which deter harmful invaders. Moreover, these friendly skin microbes can boost our own defences by prompting our skin cells to produce antimicrobial peptides, which are tiny proteins known for their pathogen-fighting properties. We'll discuss antimicrobial peptides in greater detail in Chapter 14.

Similar protective mechanisms are also at work in our

upper respiratory tract, which includes our noses and throats. The microbes residing in these parts play a crucial role in ensuring that harmful disease-causing microbes don't move down to the lungs and potentially cause infections. Friendly microbes also harmonize our immune response.

Studies on mice have shown that their native respiratory microbes influence how various immune cells and antibodies react to flu virus infections. When these mice were given antibiotics, their flu symptoms worsened. Disrupting the natural balance of microbes in the throat can also lead to increased colonization by potentially harmful bacteria. Similarly, some studies suggest that people who have taken antibiotics might be more susceptible to upper respiratory infections. And children who had certain bacteria in their noses were less likely to get ear infections, especially if they had not taken antibiotics recently.

Antibiotics can also harm us through the microbes they don't target. Certain disease-causing microbes are naturally unaffected by antibiotics even without resistance genes because antibiotics impact different bacteria differently. Some bacteria don't need to acquire resistance because the antibiotics weren't meant for them in the first place. These bacteria can multiply rapidly when competing bacteria are reduced by antibiotic treatment.

Infections are also caused by microbes other than bacteria. When you take an antibiotic for a viral or fungal infection, not only is the drug ineffective for what ails you, but it might also make it easier for disease-causing microbes to flourish. Take, for example, fungi. Many fungi live harmoniously in parts of our body, including our skin, mouth and gut. But when antibiotics clear out beneficial bacteria, fungi can overgrow, leading to yeast infections and oral thrush. *Candida albicans* is one such fungus that can cause an infection when its bacterial neighbours are diminished.

The good news is that once a course of antibiotics ends, the body's microbial community typically begins to rebound. It often resembles its original state within a few weeks of stopping the medicines. Still, while many bacteria might rebound, certain ones might remain reduced in numbers or even disappear altogether. And repeated courses of antibiotics seem to make it harder for a healthy microbiome to bounce back each time. The way these microbes function might also change. For example, a person might end up with a different set of bacteria than they had before, which can impact the overall health of the gut. This altered state of the microbiome can last for several months or possibly longer.

My goal in mentioning these unintended consequences of antibiotic use is not to put anyone off antibiotics altogether. No one is arguing about the legitimate, judicious use of antibiotics. But as an informed user, you should know about how drugs impact your health. It's not just your community or country at risk here – it's your own body.

9

How We Stumbled on Antibiotics (and Resistance)

Before Antibiotics and Antibacterial Drugs

While antibiotics as we know them have been around for less than a hundred years, our ancestors used early, crude forms of antibiotics. Researchers have found traces of tetracycline, a commonly used antibiotic today, in human skeletons dating back to 350–550 CE in Sudanese Nubia. What makes tetracyclines particularly fascinating is their ability to bond with the mineral portions of bones and tooth enamel and leave permanent marks of their existence. This offers us a rare and intriguing glimpse into the health practices of ancient civilizations.

And it's not just bones that tell this story. In Jordan, local red soils known for their healing properties have been found to contain antibiotic-producing bacteria. These produced substances like actinomycin C2 and actinomycin C3, which have properties similar to antibiotic used in modern medicine.

Modern microbiology has existed for less than two centuries and so people in antiquity did not know what microbes were or what they looked like. But they had stumbled on an amazing class of organisms – fungi and soil bacteria – which, to this day, contribute the vast majority of antibiotics in use.

The Greeks and Romans believed in the healing properties of fungi, especially mushrooms. They also valued moulds that developed on bread and other perishables for their curative effects. For example, the renowned Greek physician Hippocrates recognized the medicinal benefits of fungi, particularly yeast, to address specific gynaecological issues. Around the same time, the Roman scholar Pliny the Elder, in his magnum opus *Historia Naturalis*, devoted an entire chapter to detailing the remedial qualities of mushrooms.

However, in Europe in the Middle Ages, such profound insights into the curative powers of mould and fungi faded, and the emphasis shifted to more bizarre treatments such as magic stones, potions, and rituals. Yet, the belief in the therapeutic abilities of mould was not entirely forgotten across the globe. Far from Europe, in the Americas, the Mayans were renowned for their advanced understanding of astronomy and mathematics. They used a fungus named 'cuxum' that thrived on roasted green corn left untouched for some time, and this was their treatment for ulcers and infections of the intestines.

Additionally, even after the advent of modern microbiology, several communities swore by the healing powers of moulds. The Ukrainians, Yugoslavs, and populations in rural Greece used bread mould as a remedy for injuries well into the 1900s. They believed that as remedies, moulds were more potent than burgeoning pharmaceutical offerings.

Microbiology would not exist without the microscope, and for this invention, we must thank a Dutch draper and lens grinder. Antoni van Leeuwenhoek peered into the microscopic world for the first time in 1675 with his self-crafted microscope, which was nothing like its modern descendant. His microscope was a mere magnifying glass affixed to a brass piece measuring three inches. But even with this primitive technology, he revealed a world that had so far been unseen. Within a droplet of his saliva, he noticed minuscule entities that appeared to be in motion. The revelation that tiny creatures resided within his body was staggering, awe-inspiring, and unnerving all at the same time. Referring to them as 'little animals', he estimated them to be a thousandfold smaller than a louse's eye. And biology would never be the same again.

Let's fast forward to the 1830s. By then, the microscope had seen many generations of design improvements. In the nineteenth century, the compound microscope transformed the microbiologist's ability to perceive the unseen world of microscopic organisms. This advanced device revealed countless single-celled, rod-shaped entities inhabiting not just our bodies but every conceivable space. Their rod-like shape inspired their naming: 'bacteria', from the Greek word for stick or staff.

The field of medicine was now emerging from conjecture and dogma to a true scientific discipline, and many medical advancements were built on these early scientific discoveries. For example, in 1865, Joseph Lister, an English surgeon, introduced the concept of using antiseptics in surgical procedures. Inspired by the work of French chemist and microbiologist Louis Pasteur, who had shown that the microorganisms in the air led to fermentation and putrefaction, he aimed to reduce the high incidences of post-surgical wound infections. Lister believed that these microbes were also responsible for causing infections in wounds. He was convinced that the air in medical environments needed to be disinfected to prevent infections, proposing that a barrier could be used to shield wounds from the surrounding air. His hypothesis was grounded in the belief that all diseases might be preventable by eliminating airborne germs through filtration, heat, or chemical means.

Lister put his theory into practice using carbolic acid as an antiseptic to treat compound fractures. By applying a pad dipped in carbolic acid to wounds and later using a lotion form directly on wounds during surgery, he observed a significant reduction in infection rates. This seemingly simple addition drastically reduced post-surgery fatality rates, which until then were hovering around a terrifying 50 per cent. Before Lister's work, despite successful surgeries, patients often succumbed to subsequent infections. 'The operation was successful, but the patient died' was often a simple statement of fact rather than a sarcastic comment.

Lister's methods, shared through articles in *The Lancet* and in presentations to the medical community, led to changes in surgical practice, such as the use of clean gloves, the washing of hands with antiseptic solutions, and the use of non-porous materials for instrument handles. His pioneering work laid the groundwork for the modern use of aseptic techniques in surgery, making operative procedures markedly safer and transforming the landscape of medical practice.

By the latter part of the nineteenth century, Louis Pasteur had made microbiology a true scientific discipline. In 1877, he noticed that deadly organisms, when rendered harmless, could ward off infections. This landmark discovery shed light on the potential of immunity against a slew of infectious diseases. However, during this era, death from bacterial infections was still rampant, with bacteria exhibiting the ability to rapidly multiply in the bloodstream or exacerbate even the tiniest wounds.

It was Robert Koch, a German bacteriologist, who would later refine the understanding of these minuscule invaders. In 1880, he posited a radical idea: microorganisms weren't merely consequences of diseases but were, in fact, their very cause. In collaboration with Friedrich Loeffler, Koch laid down a set of ground rules that changed the way we understood diseases. Finally, scientists could become detectives investigating infectious diseases and revealing their mysterious causes. These rules, known as Koch's Postulates, were a checklist to confirm if microbes, like bacteria, were the culprits behind a disease. By setting out a clear path to follow, these guidelines helped scientists pin the root causes of diseases such as cholera and TB.

Any discussion about infectious diseases is incomplete without charting the early history of vaccines. Did you know that vaccines actually preceded the modern discovery of antibiotics by over one hundred years? The advent of vaccination marked a pivotal shift in medical history, and hundreds of millions of lives have been saved since.

In 1796, in the English countryside, physician Edward Jenner found that those inoculated with cowpox exhibited immunity to the deadly viral disease smallpox. This discovery brought hope to countless individuals since smallpox had claimed millions of lives at that point.

The groundwork for this idea, however, was laid by Jenner's many predecessors, among them the fearless Lady Mary Wortley Montagu. With the flair of an eighteenth-century influencer, Montagu brought 'variolation' to attention of European high society after witnessing its efficacy in Turkey. Variolation involved a deliberate exposure to smallpox in a controlled manner. Despite a 2 per cent mortality rate, it offered a significant reduction in the risk posed by the disease as compared to natural infection. By choosing to variolate her own children, Montagu not only showed personal conviction but also set a trend that would finally receive royal endorsement.

Jenner, standing on the shoulders of these variolation practices, recognized the potential in milkmaids' resistance to smallpox after a cowpox infection. The critical experiment that would anchor Jenner's legacy involved the young James Phipps. In a procedure that would be deemed highly risky by today's standards, Jenner transferred pus from a cowpox lesion into cuts on Phipps's arm, later challenging the boy's immune response with smallpox material. Phipps's survival without contracting the disease was a monumental success. Jenner's initial attempts to disseminate his findings were met with caution and resistance by the scientific elite of the Royal Society, but his determination to share his discovery led him to bypass traditional channels and self-publish his results.

From infection prevention, let's move on to treatment. Chemotherapy was a breakthrough in treating infections using drugs, and it refers to the use of drugs to treat diseases by killing or inhibiting the growth of the causative agents. While the term is widely used today for treating cancer cells, it's early and broad application was in the design of antibacterials, which were chemicals that stop bacterial infections.

Strictly speaking, antibiotics are distinguished from human antibacterials in that they are made naturally by other microbes. Antibacterials are created in the laboratory and until the discovery of antibiotics, they were the primary ways to treat bacterial infections. From antibacterials we will move on to antibiotics.

Salvarsan

The story of antibiotics, the invisible shields that protect us from bacterial invasions, has been a journey of hits, misses, and adaptations. Treating bacterial infections started with a dream – the vision of a 'magic bullet' that would specifically target disease-causing microbes without harming the host. This was the vision of one man, Paul Ehrlich, in the early twentieth century, and came following his intriguing observations with aniline dyes and bacteria. Ehrlich's groundbreaking work laid the cornerstone for modern drug discovery. The first systematic approach to vanquishing a disease-causing bacterium was made in the early twentieth century by him. He experimented with Salvarsan, a drug developed to treat syphilis, a disease that until then had been considered incurable.

Ehrlich, alongside his colleagues Alfred Bertheim and Sahachiro Hata, conducted extensive research into the properties of hundreds of synthesized chemical compounds before finally achieving success with Compound 606, which was subsequently named Salvarsan. This is a synthetic arsenic drug that proved effective in treating the early and middle stages of syphilis. The mechanism by which Salvarsan eradicated the bacteria responsible for the disease was not understood at the time, yet it managed to do so without harming the patients.

Salvarsan wasn't perfect – its injections were tedious, and it had side effects. However, it became the world's most prescribed drug until penicillin, the first bona fide antibiotic, dethroned it in the 1940s. Ehrlich's groundbreaking contributions were acknowledged globally when he was honoured with the Nobel Prize in Physiology or Medicine in 1908, and Salvarsan became widely available in 1910.

In 1913, Marconi Transatlantic Wireless Telegraph's breathless report was published in the *New York Times* from London and gives us a flavour of how popular the man was:

> Prof. Paul Ehrlich's address overshadowed all other events in the International Medical Congress today. He is a small man of frail build, with thin white hair bordering a peaked skull cap, and with alert eyes set in a pale, rather featureless face terminating in a tiny, pointed beard. He wore a dusty frock coat, and his voice was shrill rather than powerful. Such was the savant whom thousands of his fellows greeted with the sort of cheering that men grant to a hero.

In his later years, Ehrlich delved deep into the study of

tumours, exploring the relationship between two types of cancers: sarcomas and carcinomas. Sarcomas are rare cancers that start in the body's connective tissues, like bone or muscle, while carcinomas are more common and begin in the skin or tissue linings of organs, such as the lungs or breasts. Ehrlich suggested that sarcomas might develop from carcinomas, an idea that investigated how different cancers could be related. Ehrlich's hypothesis was an innovative idea in cancer research at the time, but modern science views these two cancer types as uniquely different due to their origins and characteristics.

A biography by Ehrlich's former secretary Martha Marquardt paints an intimate picture of his life in Frankfurt, where the street housing his institute was named Paul Ehrlichstrasse in his honour. However, due to the persecutions during the Nazi era, because of Ehrlich's Jewish heritage, the name was changed. After the Second World War, Polish authorities renamed his birthplace Strehlen as Ehrlichstadt as a fitting tribute to the scientific pioneer.

Prontosil

Shortly after Ehrlich's discovery, German pathologist Gerhard Domagk discovered prontosil, a sulfonamide drug potent enough to save his daughter from having her limbs amputated. Interestingly, this was a precursor to the drug sulfanilamide, which already existed in the dye industry. This made it unpatentable, leading to a cascade of sulfonamide derivatives. Unfortunately, these medications also led to one of the first mass cases of drug resistance, a dark omen of what was to come.

But let's go back to the story of the discovery of the antibacterial drug. In 1932, in a small laboratory in Wuppertal, Germany, Domagk was on the cusp of a scientific breakthrough. Domagk was a man haunted by memories of suffering. He had seen the devastation wrought by infectious diseases first-hand as a young medic in the trenches of First World War and later in the cholera hospitals of Russia. He had witnessed the grim realities of amputations and gas gangrene, and of medical procedures that did more harm than good because the healthcare system simply had no weapons against bacterial infections.

Years later, as he peered through his microscope at the chemical compound in front of him, he wondered, 'Could this red dyestuff, prontosil, finally offer humankind a weapon against bacterial killers?'

Domagk's work had already shown promise – mice and rabbits infected with lethal doses of bacteria had been saved by prontosil. But these animals weren't human beings, and just as Domagk began to ponder the leap from animal to human trials, fate forced his hand. His own daughter fell gravely ill with a streptococcal infection. Doctors were helpless. The heart-wrenching scenes from his past experiences now played out in his very home. Consumed by a father's desperation and a scientist's reasoning, Domagk administered a dose of prontosil to his daughter. As days passed, a miracle unfolded – she recovered fully.

Yet, Domagk was a man of rigorous scientific temperament. He refrained from publicly proclaiming his personal triumph, opting instead to wait for clinical validation. By 1935, reports from physicians who had tested prontosil began pouring in, and these were overwhelmingly positive. Domagk's discovery had given medicine a new class of weapons – antibacterial drugs based on sulfanilamide, which would save countless lives in the years to come.

In 1939, Gerhard Domagk was awarded the Nobel Prize in Physiology or Medicine, a monumental achievement, but one tinged with political complexity as he initially had to decline the award due to the political climate in Germany at the time and the onset of the Second World War. In 1947, however, following the collapse of Nazi Germany, he was formally presented with the Nobel diploma.

Penicillin

While these discoveries of chemical compounds were monumental, they were overshadowed by the serendipitous discovery of penicillin in 1928 by Alexander Fleming. This is widely considered the first true antibiotic to be discovered. Fleming stumbled upon a mould that seemed to possess antibacterial qualities, and the rest, as they say, is history. Or so the story goes – but there's actually much more to it.

How We Stumbled on Antibiotics (and Resistance)

There are many instances in science where everyone who contributed to a major advance didn't get equal credit. A very notable example is the journey that transformed penicillin from a microbiological discovery into a usable antibiotic that saved lives. Fleming's contribution is well known, in part due to an excellent public relations campaign mounted by his backers. In 1928, at St Mary's Hospital in London, Fleming returned from his summer vacation in Scotland to dirty petri dishes with colonies of the bacterium *Staphylococcus aureus*, but which also had a zone where it did not grow. Curious, Fleming examined the dishes and found that they had been contaminated by a mould named *Penicillium notatum*.

Fleming repeated his experiments and named the unknown compound in the mould that prevented growth, penicillin. But how did the world go from that basic discovery to the actual drugs that fight bacterial infections? Eric Lax recounts the story and reapportions the credit for the miracle drug in his book, *The Mould in Dr Florey's Coat*. It's a great book that highlights how it takes many people over many years to take a discovery in the lab and turn it into an actual drug.

The story of the accidental discovery of penicillin by Alexander Fleming can be narrated by schoolchildren around the world. But it took twelve years from that discovery to the production of the drug that revolutionized modern medicine. So, why did it take so long? Fleming had neither the laboratory to grow large amounts of the fungus, nor the chemical knowledge to isolate the active compound, penicillin. In fact,

Fleming did very little research on penicillin after his initial discoveries. He slowed his research on penicillin in 1931 and offered to send his mould to anyone else who wished to carry the work further.

Howard Florey, Ernst Chain, and Normal Heatley, all scientists at Oxford University, realized the potential of penicillin, and they took the baton from Fleming. It was actually Chain who first spotted Fleming's article while looking through old medical journals. The three scientists figured out the best way to grow the mould so that it would yield the most antibiotic, how to separate penicillin from the mould, and how to scale up its use as a viable drug. And in doing so, they had more to do with the use of penicillin as a drug than the discoverer himself.

In 1940, a police constable named Albert Alexander became a test case for the medical use of penicillin. There are multiple versions of how Alexander developed an infection, but the most popular account goes something like this. While working in his rose garden, he scratched his face. The scratch was infected, and Alexander suffered for months as the bacteria spread and abscesses developed on his face and arms. Having all but given up hope, doctors gave Alexander penicillin. Within a day, Alexander began to recover.

But in a cruel twist of fate, Alexander's life would depend on getting more penicillin. At that time, penicillin was so scarce that the urine of those being treated was collected. The body does not break down all the penicillin that is administered and so it can be isolated and repurified from urine and injected. But even the trace amounts that could be repurified from Alexander's urine were not enough. When the penicillin finally ran out, Alexander succumbed to his infection.

Frustrated with the lack of facilities in wartime Britain, Florey and Heatley travelled to Peoria, Illinois, the following year, crossing the Atlantic in a blacked-out airplane to avoid detection by wartime enemy forces. In the US, they worked with other scientists to purify and scale up the production of penicillin.

The original fungus species that Fleming had isolated did not yield enough penicillin to be commercially viable, and scientists kept looking for new sources. In fact, a massive 2,000 litres of Fleming's *P. notatum* was required to get enough penicillin to treat just one person.

The need for antibiotics was recognized then, just as the need for vaccines and drugs for COVID-19 was during the coronavirus pandemic. In fact, the US government pushed drug companies to work together to make adequate amounts of penicillin. In 1942, Merck and E.R. Squibb and Sons agreed to share their research, and later that year, Charles Pfizer and Company joined them.

The breakthrough only came in 1943. Kenneth Raper and his team at the Northern Regional Research Laboratory worked long hours every day growing thousands of strains of moulds. They were searching for just the right one that would yield enough of the wonder drug. One of the people entrusted with finding new sources of mould was Mary Hunt, also known as 'Mouldy Mary'. In one version of the story recounted by Eric Lax in his book, Hunt bought some musk melon (also known as cantaloupe in the US) at a market in Peoria. She recounted later that the cantaloupe had a 'pretty golden mould'. (There are other accounts that dispute Mary Hunt's side of the story, but it is likely that she did have a role in the discovery.)

This mould was identified as *Penicillium chrysogenum*, and it yielded 200 times more penicillin than Fleming's species. Further mutating the strain by using X-rays, scientists were able to increase the yield to 1,000 times the amount obtained from the original Fleming strain. And so, that mouldy fruit became the source of most of the penicillin available in the world. By 1945, a million people had been treated with penicillin. From that point on, penicillin went from being a mould with odd properties to a scarce resource and then to a mass-produced lifesaver, highlighting the global nature of scientific innovation and cooperation.

The Second World War provided the backdrop for the meteoric rise of penicillin. The drug was mass produced and saved thousands of soldiers' lives, fulfilling Paul Ehrlich's vision of a 'magic bullet' that could target pathogens without harming the host. By 1944, penicillin was available to the general public, and it seemed like humanity had finally gained the upper hand against bacterial infections.

Another breakthrough came when the brilliant British crystallographer Dorothy Hodgkin figured out what penicillin looked like in 1945, setting the stage for chemists to modify the core of the penicillin molecule to create derivatives that were even more powerful against disease-causing agents.

Fleming, Florey, and Chain were awarded the Nobel Prize in Physiology or Medicine in 1945, and Heatley was a notable omission from the honour. Hodgkin was awarded the Nobel Prize in Chemistry in 1964. Today, if you ask anyone about penicillin, they will likely remember only Fleming's name. But few people today know about Mary Hunt or about the mouldy fruit that revolutionized twentieth-century medical science.

Fleming did sound the alarm about antibiotic resistance in his 1945 Nobel Prize acceptance speech. Only a few years after the introduction of penicillin, resistant strains of *Staphylococcus aureus* began to appear in hospitals. Fleming understood that natural mutations would inevitably produce bacteria resistant to antibiotics, but even he could not foresee the scale of the problem that lay ahead.

The first wave of antibiotics was the bounty of nature like penicillin, derived mainly from moulds and soil bacteria. Chemists like John Sheehan went on a quest to synthesize penicillin from scratch, a feat that was finally achieved in the late 1950s. Sheehan's work opened the door to modifying existing antibiotics to combat resistance. As a result, methicillin was introduced in 1960 as a modified version of penicillin resistant to the penicillinase enzymes that bacteria had developed to withstand the effects of penicillin. The *New York Times* celebrated its efficacy in 1961 when it saved actor Elizabeth Taylor from a penicillin-resistant infection.

But this triumph was short-lived. By 1962, methicillin-resistant *Staphylococcus aureus* (MRSA) had already emerged. The bacteria had adapted yet again, this time by changing the protein that methicillin targeted. MRSA became a global concern, especially in hospitals, and by the 1970s and 1980s, the pace of new antibiotic discovery had slowed considerably.

By the early 2000s, more than half the *Staphylococcus aureus* cases in US hospitals were MRSA superbugs. And in the early 1990s, a more virulent strain of MRSA began circulating in various communities, affecting even healthy individuals.

Streptomycin

The groundwork laid by these pioneers paved the way for Selman Waksman's focused inquiry into microbes in the late 1930s. It was Waksman who coined the term 'antibiotic', later writing that it was a name 'I suggested in 1941 for chemical substances of microbial origin'.

Waksman proved to be a masterful detective in identifying streptomycetes, which were filamentous, Gram-positive bacteria commonly found in soil and prodigious antibiotic factories. His explorations gave us neomycin and streptomycin, the latter being a milestone in TB treatment. Waksman tapped into the strategy of producing antibiotics to outdo their microbial rivals.

In 1910, Selman Waksman made the pivotal journey from Ukraine, which was then under Russian rule, to New Jersey in the US where his family had already settled. The subsequent year, he took up undergraduate studies at Rutgers College, which was located close by. Waksman's research prowess did not go unnoticed at Rutgers, and his professor, Jacob Lipman, suggested that he devote his senior year to a comprehensive exploration of soil microbes. The findings of this year-long project were presented at the Annual Meeting of the Society of American Bacteriologists and published in the inaugural volume of the *Journal of Bacteriology*.

After that, Waksman completed a master's degree on actinomycetes. These filamentous soil bacteria, known for their sluggish growth, had long been ignored by the scientific community. This fascination particularly deepened with *Actinomyces griseus*, which had been discovered a few years earlier. It later emerged as the foundation of his future research. Waksman's work was pivotal in renaming the bacteria to *Streptomyces griseus*. With a collection of actinomycetes, he then went to the University of California in Berkeley and completed his doctoral research. And once he was done, he joined the faculty of Rutgers' Agricultural School back in New Jersey.

One of Waksman's prominent early students was Robert

Starkey. Originally mentored by Waksman during his doctoral studies, Starkey subsequently transformed into a collaborative researcher and fellow educator. The duo, along with an ever-growing team of doctoral students led by Waksman, dedicated years to pioneering research on soil microbiology, laying the foundation for various studies on antibiotics.

In a seminal paper published in *Soil Science* in 1923, Waksman and Starkey stumbled on antibiotics without appreciating their significance. They found that certain actinomycetes exhibited an intriguing behaviour – while growing, they inhibited the growth of other bacteria in the soil. In their article, they wrote, 'Certain actinomycetes produce substances toxic to bacteria ... around an actinomycete colony, upon a plate, a zone is found free from bacterial growth.'

These findings hinted at the possibility that these actinomycetes might be producing substances – which would come to be known as antibiotics – that could combat human pathogens. This connection was missed by everyone who read the scientific article and even by Waksman himself. Had this realization struck earlier, perhaps the credit for discovering the first antibiotic would have landed with Waksman rather than with Fleming!

In 1937, Waksman experienced an epiphany. He remembered his earlier observations with Starkey about microbial interactions in the soil. He gave his doctoral students the task of studying these interactions in a controlled laboratory environment, observing how mixed bacterial cultures interacted, and possibly inhibited one another. Their efforts bore fruit, yielding antibiotics like actinomycin, streptothricin, fumigacin, and clavacin. Yet, as groundbreaking as these were, each of these antibiotics was found to be toxic to laboratory animals, presenting a serious challenge in their application in human health. Surely there would be an antibiotic that would be safe to use in people?

The breakthrough came when Albert Schatz joined Waksman's team as a doctoral student. Though his career was briefly interrupted by military service, Schatz screened soil samples under Waksman's guidance. On his eleventh attempt at soil plating from Rutgers Agriculture School's farm soil, he managed to isolate a strain of *Streptomyces griseus* with antibiotic properties. This newfound antibiotic was named 'streptomycin' by Waksman and Schatz, and soon studies confirmed that streptomycin was safe to use in both laboratory animals and humans.

Sensing the potential of streptomycin to treat TB, Waksman collaborated with the Mayo Clinic to test the antibiotic. The results were revolutionary: for the first time, there was an antibiotic able to treat tuberculosis. Accolades came quickly to the senior scientist, and Waksman won the Nobel Prize in Physiology or Medicine in 1952, but his doctoral student, Schatz, did not.

Tensions erupted between Waksman and Schatz, concerning the distribution of royalties from the sales of streptomycin. At the outset, 80 per cent of the funds were earmarked for the establishment of a novel microbiological research initiative at Rutgers. Meanwhile, Waksman had laid claim to the remaining 20 per cent of royalties, channelling them primarily towards extending streptomycin research beyond Rutgers.

However, the distribution of royalties was soon recalibrated. Waksman, in light of his significant commitment to the streptomycin project, was accorded a portion of the royalties as additional compensation over his regular university salary. This led to unforeseen legal strife as Schatz sought legal remedy. The impending court battle, however, never came to pass. A settlement was negotiated outside of court, with Schatz assenting to a proposal presented by Waksman.

Waksman proposed a distribution of 10 per cent of the royalties among twenty-six individuals, including students and laboratory employees. Schatz, credited with discovering the streptomycin-producing culture, would receive the lion's share. Schatz was also subsequently conferred with several accolades, including the Rutgers Medal, by the university. During the commemoration of the fiftieth anniversary of the discovery of streptomycin, he delivered lectures at Rutgers. And following student demand, a plaque recognizing him as a co-discoverer of streptomycin was affixed at the site of its discovery.

An editorial perspective in *The Lancet Infectious Diseases* in 2005 delved into the controversy. The point of contention wasn't the discovery itself – streptomycin's value was beyond doubt. The journal noted, however, that 'in a paternalistic era when credit tended to go to the head of department, the Nobel Committee made a considerable mistake by failing to recognise Schatz's contribution'. According to an account by a former student, Waksman was hurt by the lawsuit by Schatz. Obviously, he could not be held responsible for the omission by the Nobel committee.

Though streptomycin was the first medicine used to treat TB, its use is not as common now because more bacteria have become resistant to it, and it has to be given by injection.

Waksman's most lasting contribution, however, is the method he developed to identify and test for new antibiotics from soil bacteria. A recent scientific review in the *Journal of Antibiotics* has found that 90 per cent of the medically useful antibiotics in use today come from the soil bacteria that Waksman devoted his life to studying – the actinomycetes!

In addition, a commentary written by microbiologist Kim Lewis in *Nature* over a decade ago urged microbiologists to bring back Waksman's method to test the vast community of soil bacteria that had not yet been screened for antibiotics. Lewis wrote: 'We need to revive the Waksman platform. We stopped discovering useful classes of antibiotics from soil bacteria decades ago, but that was during a time when it was impossible to culture more than 99 per cent of bacterial species. Today, methods to culture these microbes are being developed, providing access to chemical diversity that was previously missed.'

Another antibiotic that came from soil samples was vancomycin. Isolated in 1953 from a soil sample from the jungles of Borneo, vancomycin was initially plagued by impurities, leading to its discoverers at the pharmaceutical company Eli Lilly and Company to nickname it 'Mississippi mud'. But despite these early challenges, the drug was refined and entered clinical use in the 1960s, primarily as an intravenous treatment. Remarkably, it remained largely effective against bacterial infections until the mid-1980s, a longevity attributed to its restricted use in hospital settings.

The late 1970s marked a turning point in antibiotic resistance. In Europe, a drug related to vancomycin known as avoparcin was approved for use in agriculture, enabling the emergence of vancomycin resistance. At the same time, in the US, due to a major MRSA outbreak, the use of the drug vancomycin increased massively, jumping 100 times over the next twenty years. This surge in use, both in agriculture and healthcare, set the stage for the emergence of vancomycin-resistant superbugs.

Mobile resistance

At first, physicians would often prescribe antibiotics even when there was only a small chance of a bacterial infection just to be safe. But as antibiotics became widely used, bacteria that could resist these drugs started to appear, leading to diminished effectiveness of antibiotic treatment.

How We Stumbled on Antibiotics (and Resistance)

In the 1950s, Japanese scientist Tsutomu Watanabe found strains of *Shigella dysenteriae* that were resistant to multiple antibiotics. Then in the 1960s, he made the striking observation that antibiotic resistance could spread among bacteria. In a 1963 article in the journal *Bacteriology Reviews*, working with Japanese colleagues, he called the spread of antibiotic resistance an example of 'infective heredity'.

The backdrop to this groundbreaking Japanese research was the aftermath of the Second World War, which was marked by a surge in cases of bacillary dysentery. While factors like post-war dislocation, poverty, and deterioration of health services likely compounded the issue, the primary culprit remained *Shigella dysenteriae*. Medical practitioners initially relied on sulfa drugs to counteract the bacterium, but as it developed resistance, they shifted to newer antibiotics, including streptomycin and tetracycline.

However, by 1953, certain *Shigella dysenteriae* strains had become resistant to these drugs as well. Interestingly, while each strain became resistant to one specific drug, it remained vulnerable to others. A critical turn of events occurred in 1955 when a Japanese woman returning from Hong Kong displayed symptoms of dysentery. Upon examination, a strain of *Shigella dysenteriae* from her infection was shown to possess resistance to several antibiotics. Following this, Japan was besieged by numerous dysentery outbreaks caused by *Shigella dysenteriae* strains resistant to four different kinds of antibiotics.

Even more alarming was the realization that such resistance was not restricted to *Shigella*. Certain *E. coli* cultures, sourced from patients who had infections with resistant strains of *Shigella dysenteriae*, exhibited exactly the same patterns of resistance. This hinted at the possibility that there had been genetic exchange between *E. coli* and *Shigella dysenteriae*, with resistance genes traversing horizontally. In a sense, this would be like humans exchanging coveted trading cards. Soon, this phenomenon was confirmed across various bacteria, and today we know that it is one of the primary drivers of superbug emergence.

But what was this elusive set of genes that effortlessly transgressed boundaries? In pursuit of an answer, Watanabe and his colleague Toshio Fukasawa theorized the presence of a distinct genetic entity floating freely within bacterial cells and not tethered to the primary chromosome. These snippets of DNA would replicate independently and would encode traits beneficial during emergencies.

Watanabe's 1963 article in *Bacteriology Reviews* affirmed that resistance to streptomycin and the other three antibiotics was encoded on just such an entity. This genetic structure facilitated the swift transfer of multiple antibiotic resistance genes. Today, Watanabe's mobile genetic elements are known as plasmids.

In 1992, Stuart Levy, one of Watanabe's students, wrote *The Antibiotic Paradox*, and in this landmark book, he highlighted the double-edged nature of antibiotics. While on the one hand antibiotics revolutionized human health, on the other, they inadvertently bolstered bacterial resistance, leading to superbugs evolving to counteract these challenges.

Reflecting on the work of Watanabe, Levy acknowledged the discovery of resistance genes that could be transferred through mobile packets 'opened the eyes of microbiologists and medical scientists to a breadth of gene spread never before imagined'.

The era of superbugs was well under way.

10

Drowning in Antibiotics

The Patancheru Industrial Area near Hyderabad in India is a centre for the bulk production of drugs. It is here that an international team of scientists made a startling discovery in 2009. The wastewater from the local treatment plant, responsible for processing effluents from dozens of drug manufacturers, contained extraordinarily high levels of antibiotics and other drugs. The levels of one antibiotic, ciprofloxacin in the industrial wastewater were so high that it was like pouring a full litre bottle of medicine into a small pond. And while this is lower than a dose that might be prescribed to a human, no one knows for sure what the long-term effects of exposure to these drugs might be.

Even more troubling, these contaminants weren't only confined to the plant. They flowed downstream into other rivers, affecting larger geographical regions. The waters of

Patancheru had turned into a cocktail of antibiotics, and people were consuming them without being aware of their presence.

In one set of incidents in Patancheru, pharmaceutical companies were reported to have dumped around fifty kilograms of the antibiotic ciprofloxacin into rivers daily. This resulted in river sediment downstream containing close to a milligram of the antibiotic per gram of organic matter.

On an immediate level, this environmental contamination creates the perfect circumstances for antibiotic resistance to spread rapidly among bacteria. What's even more concerning is that after environmental bacteria acquire these resistance genes, they can pass them along to bacteria that interact with humans and animals. This could be the breeding ground for the next MDR superbug.

If this antibiotic contamination were an isolated incident, it would be troubling enough. Yet, a separate scientific study painted a similarly grim picture for the Yamuna river, the lifeline for a large swathe of northern India. This river supplies potable water to millions in one of the country's most densely populated regions.

Researchers took samples from various points along its course, including hospitals, residential areas, and drug manufacturing facilities, across different seasons to understand the scope of the problem. What they found was disturbing: antibiotic concentrations spiked notably during the pre-monsoon season, with drugs like ofloxacin, amoxicillin, and erythromycin showing up in measurable amounts.

Ever since antibiotics have been produced on a mass scale for human use, they have polluted the environment in many ways – through human waste, the improper disposal of unused medications, agricultural runoff, rampant use in domestic animal farming, and waste from antibiotic manufacturing.

But there's yet another concern. Microbes play an indispensable role in maintaining ecosystem health. The introduction of antibiotics in the environment disrupts microbial communities, altering their biological make-up.

Although environmental concentrations of antibiotics are usually lower than those needed to slow bacterial growth or kill bacteria directly, the presence of antibiotics can select for resistant strains. It is plausible to think that contaminating antibiotics and resistant bacteria can move up the food chain. For example, plants and crops might be able to absorb antibiotics and resistant bacteria from contaminated soil and water. Animals consuming these plants might accumulate antibiotics and harbour resistant bacteria.

One of the more insidious aspects of this issue is how easily it can be overlooked. Since antibiotics are considered safe for human consumption, they often fly under the radar as environmental hazards. This raises a disconcerting question: where else might antibiotic pollution be occurring while we remain entirely unaware of it?

There's a solution to this issue, though it requires a lot

of coordination. Communities, pharmaceutical industry stakeholders, and regulatory agencies can come together to monitor the looming threat of this invisible pollution. Framing of regulations, public awareness of the issue, and joint monitoring can help mitigate antibiotic pollution. In addition, a more comprehensive and nuanced understanding of the scale and implications of antibiotic pollution should be a priority.

Factories that manufacture antibiotics inadvertently contribute to the problem, but finding a direct link between environmental pollutants and the spread of resistance can sometimes be difficult. The fact is that antibiotic resistance is a puzzle with many missing pieces. It isn't just antibiotics in the environment that speed up the spread of resistance. Other chemicals in our environment, such as metals used in biological agents in agriculture, can also help select for antibiotic resistance, as can disinfectants and solvents.

Water is also undoubtedly a primary source for the spread of resistant bacteria and antibiotics. Water that is contaminated, by human and animal waste, and industrial and agricultural runoff, can end up being used in irrigation, consumed directly by animals and even by humans. Most routine tests of water quality in India do not check for the presence of antibiotics at reasonable concentrations. And depending on where you live, there might well be antibiotics in the water that you use every day.

Antibiotics leak into various aquatic ecosystems. While it

is almost certain that their concentration in drinking water, for example, would be too low to cause the acceleration of resistance, there might be hotspots where antibiotic levels are very high, like at sewage treatment plants and points directly downstream of pharmaceutical manufacturing plants. Such areas show stronger evidence of driving resistance. Here, not only do concentrations significantly exceed levels known to induce resistance, but the presence of resistant bacteria and antibiotic resistance genes also increases markedly.

The use of the manure of animals treated with antibiotics as a fertilizer has also been linked to increased resistance in farmlands. Although it's challenging to definitively attribute these superbugs to the antibiotics in manure, some studies have demonstrated that added antibiotics add evolutionary pressure on specific bacterial strains to acquire resistance.

But industrial waste isn't our only challenge. When people take antibiotics, not all of them are used by the body, and the surplus is released in our urine and stool. In prosperous countries with good sewage systems, these antibiotics might be filtered out, but antibiotics will elsewhere still slip through. There might be tiny amounts of antibiotics in sewage systems, but these can accumulate over time.

In areas with inadequate resources for managing human and animal waste, environmental transmission can significantly worsen antibiotic resistance. The transmission route for superbugs often involves direct or indirect contact between humans and animals, most commonly through contamination via faecal matter.

The problem is especially acute where wastewater is untreated and directly discharged into rivers. The WHO estimates that about 2 billion people worldwide drink water contaminated with faeces. This poses not only the problem of getting sick with disease-causing superbugs, but also of further spread. This is clearly a vicious cycle. Greater resistance found in superbugs requires the use of more antibiotics to combat them, which leads to more production, more use, and yet more environmental discharge. All of this leads back to the environmental reservoir.

Lower-income countries face disproportionately higher concentrations of drugs in their rivers. One study found that the problem was most acute in parts of Africa and Asia. For example, Bangladesh stood out with more than 300 times the safe level of metronidazole, a drug used for certain infections, in its rivers. In Kenya, the inappropriate disposal of sewage and waste led to antibiotic concentrations that were up to 100 times of safe levels in rivers. There's a cruel irony here. The same factors that contribute to high infectious disease burdens in low-resource settings are the ones that lead to the rise of antibiotic-resistant superbugs.

Research has also shown that superbugs can spread through contaminated food or surfaces, particularly in hospitals and clinics, which are hotspots for various infectious diseases. Food items, such as raw vegetables, can also serve as vectors for the spread of resistant bacteria. While cases of foodborne illnesses linked to pathogens like *Salmonella* and *E. coli* are well documented, fewer studies have explored whether consuming contaminated produce increases the risk of carrying antibiotic-resistant bacteria. However, it's known that fresh produce often harbours various forms of resistant bacteria, necessitating the cautious utilization of human and animal waste as fertilizers in agriculture to minimize both the transmission and evolution of resistance.

A solution to combat antibiotic resistance must include proper sanitation, access to clean water, limits on non-medical use of antibiotics, and robust public health policy on the prevention of diseases and the proper use of antibiotics. Proper sanitation and disposal of sewage should be a priority since it would limit exposure to antibiotics and align with general hygiene and infection control. From a technological standpoint, basic waste treatment should also be a key priority as it would mitigate multiple risks, including those associated with antibiotic-resistant bacteria. Sewage epidemiology is still a developing field, and it received a significant boost during the COVID-19 pandemic. Similar genetic markers in wastewater would link resistance genes to the spread of superbugs in the clinic.

The exact amount of antibiotics that have been commercially produced until now is unknown. But there are conservative estimates that many millions of metric tonnes have made their way into the environment in the past few decades. There's a lot that we need to learn about the specific environmental conditions conducive to the spread of resistance genes and the emergence of superbugs. But we are making new discoveries every year.

Finding the smoking gun of a direct transmission – in other words, piecing together the link between the use of one antibiotic to the development of a superbug – is hard. There are many steps from the source to the disease. So, we rely on indirect but plausible hypotheses on the prevalence of resistance genes near places with high amounts of pollution. The evidence shows that it is possible that the transmission of resistance genes and resistant bacteria occurs from the environment to humans. Researchers have found the concentration of antibiotics and resistance genes to be directly linked to human activity nearby.

It is useful here to draw a parallel with climate change. Scientists know that there are long-term variations in climate that took place even before humans existed. But they've been able to tie the recent warming of the planet to human events since the first Industrial Revolution. No one can point to one factory or vehicle and say definitively that *this* contributed a certain portion of the change we are experiencing. However, larger trends point to human activities leading to climate change.

Similarly, the point isn't that one person popping an extra antibiotic is directly responsible for the rise of the next superbug – it's that certain human practices accelerate the process of the development and spread of resistance genes. The message is that while natural antibiotic production has been part of all our ecosystems for millennia, human activities have drastically altered the landscape, creating new challenges in the fight against superbugs.

In recent years, climate change and pollution are two factors that are now thought to play a role in the rise of superbugs. In fact, two significant studies seem to have found direct links between them. The WHO has spotlighted climate change as a potent catalyst for the emergence of infectious diseases. There has been quite a lot of attention paid to vector-borne diseases, such as malaria. After all, as the geographic range of mosquitoes increases due to a warming planet, malaria is expected to spread to new locations. The potential rise of new disease-causing microbes from the thawing Arctic ice has also been a point of scientific focus.

In May 2018, a study published in *Nature Climate Change* analysed disease-causing bacteria across forty-one states in the US to determine if antibiotic resistance was linked to any large-scale environmental factors. The results showed that both local temperature increases and rising population densities are linked to increases in antibiotic resistance in common disease-causing microbes. Specifically, the research found that a 10°Celsius rise in temperature corresponded with a resistance increase of around 4 per cent for *E. coli*, 2 per cent for *Klebsiella pneumoniae*, and 3 per cent for *Staphylococcus aureus*, which are three of our Deadly Six superbugs.

This relationship between temperature and antibiotic

resistance appears to be consistent for most antibiotic types and superbugs, and it only appears to be intensifying. Interestingly, the study found that resistance to certain antibiotics increased more with temperature change as compared to resistance to others. Why this might be the case isn't clear yet.

This is not a minor issue when considering how much hotter the world is expected to get. Some climate projections predict that parts of the US will experience a temperature surge of around 10 °Celsius by the end of the century. Assuming that the observed temperature-resistance relationship stays the same and it can be extended into the future, this would translate to an additional 10 per cent resistance for certain antibiotics.

Another dimension the study explored was population density. Areas with high-density populations can often serve as hubs for the rapid spread of resistant strains. The data underscored this notion: a rise in density akin to transitioning from the rural expanses of the US to the bustling metropolis of Boston, Massachusetts, was linked to a 6 per cent upswing in antibiotic resistance for *Klebsiella pneumoniae* and a 3 per cent increase for *E. coli*.

But what could possibly be the connection between temperature and antibiotic resistance? Unfortunately, while these studies can find correlations, they can't infer the causes. There are a few plausible hypotheses though. One is that elevated temperatures foster the transfer of plasmids through which bacteria acquire resistance genes. If temperature expedites this genetic exchange, it might accelerate the spread of resistance across bacterial populations. In addition, temperature is also known to influence how fast bacteria grow, and so a second hypothesis is that rising temperatures speed up the growth and transmission of resistance genes and superbugs.

However, these were the results of one study focusing on the US, and so we must be careful before drawing broader conclusions. Still, it's tempting to consider what the implications might be for India. The country is densely populated, and many parts of India will be subjected to rising temperatures on an unprecedented scale in the next few decades. There's potential for the problem of superbugs to get even worse.

What about pollution?

In August 2023, a study published in the *Lancet Planetary Health* journal found that particulate matter (PM) 2.5, a common air pollutant that is very harmful to health, may be a significant driver of antibiotic resistance worldwide. PM2.5 are tiny particles in the air, smaller than 2.5 micrometres in size, making them easy to breathe in.

The research analysed data from 116 countries over nearly two decades and linked the levels of PM2.5 in the air to antibiotic resistance. With data from millions of bacterial samples, they found that nearly half a million early deaths might have been due to antibiotic resistance connected with PM2.5. The authors even suggested that PM2.5 might be transporting genes responsible for antibiotic resistance across vast distances. It might also be encouraging the transfer of these resistance genes between different bacteria.

The silver lining here is that by controlling PM2.5 levels, we might have a way to combat antibiotic resistance. The study suggests that if we can bring down PM2.5 levels to the target set by the WHO, we could decrease global antibiotic resistance by almost 17 per cent. This could prevent about a quarter of the early deaths related to antibiotic resistance by the year 2050. Places like North Africa and West Asia, which suffer most from PM2.5 pollution, would particularly benefit from such efforts.

The 'One Health' approach, first put forward by various United Nations' agencies, suggests that the well-being of humans, animals, and the environment is interconnected. While previous studies largely attributed antibiotic resistance to excessive antibiotic use in humans and animals, this study tied in an environmental aspect directly.

So, what can we conclude from all of this information? It is clear that we cannot treat human health and antibiotic use in isolation any more. Human misuse of antibiotics is the greatest factor in the rise of superbugs. But we've only started to appreciate that there are also more subtle environmental factors at work. As India and the world grapple with air pollution, increasing population density, and rising local temperatures, understanding how these factors contribute to the spread of antibiotic resistance will be crucial for our future health.

11

Fat Animals and Antibiotics

As with the discovery of penicillin by Alexander Fleming in 1928, another accidental discovery in 1948 would change the course of medical history. This one occurred near the Lederle Laboratories campus in the state of New York. In the late 1940s, fishermen near the pharmaceutical company began to notice that the trout they were catching were much larger than normal. This observation made its way to biochemist Thomas Jukes, who had a hypothesis which he was about to test. And so, on a quiet Christmas Day in 1948 in the town of Pearl River, New York, he entered the halls of Lederle Laboratories with a simple mission – to weigh 133 juvenile chickens. Little did he know that this seemingly mundane task would have far-reaching implications.

This story, expertly narrated by Maryn McKenna in her book *Plucked*, occurred against the backdrop of a change that first occurred in the US and then in India. In the early twentieth century, chickens were primarily raised for eggs. However, by the 1930s, in the US, chickens became an agricultural commodity, raised by the thousands and confined indoors for meat and eggs.

With this shift, there was a growing demand for synthetic nutrition to accelerate the growth of larger chickens. This set the stage for Jukes, who became a sought-after expert in poultry nutrition, and for companies like Lederle Laboratories on the forefront of this emerging field, to gain prominence. Lederle, although primarily a pharmaceutical company, was then exploring the intersection of antibiotics and nutrition.

When Jukes joined Lederle in 1942, the race for antibiotic discovery was in full swing. Companies globally were sending out tubes, seeking samples containing potential antibiotic-producing moulds. Lederle struck gold with a sample from Missouri which contained a bacterium that produced a compound that would later be known as chlortetracycline.

Although Jukes's primary role at Lederle was in nutrition, his expertise and the company's antibiotic discoveries would soon converge. Jukes figured that the larger trout that the fishermen were finding were due to the effects of aureomycin, the antibiotic Lederle produced, in the runoff water from the campus.

Jukes's methodology was meticulous. He put the chickens on a weak diet to discern the effects of potential additives clearly. When the eggs hatched, the chicks were divided into various groups, each receiving different dietary supplements and a by-product from aureomycin production. On that fateful Christmas Day, Jukes's findings were astonishing. The chicks that received the aureomycin by-product outperformed all others, weighing significantly more. The implications of this discovery were profound. A minute amount of aureomycin, almost negligible in weight, had the potential to revolutionize poultry farming.

Jukes had inadvertently unveiled a discovery that would reshape agriculture. The ramifications extended beyond just poultry farming, influencing global trade, labour practices, and even the diets of people worldwide. Chicken is now the most popular meat in the US, India, and many other countries, and antibiotics are now regularly used as a growth enhancer.

In 1950, upon the official revelation of Jukes' discovery, the *New York Times* highlighted aureomycin's 'hitherto unsuspected nutritional powers', predicting it would wield 'enormous long-range significance for the survival of the human race'.

The introduction of antibiotics in agriculture was widespread and swift through the 1950s. However, the bliss was short-lived. What began as a promising avenue for bolstering food security soon manifested its grim side. Many scientists, including American physician and microbiologist Stuart Levy, advocated for the prudent use of antibiotics, especially in agriculture.

In a paper published in the *New England Journal of Medicine* in 1976, Levy showed that antibiotic-resistant bacteria from chickens fed antibiotic-laced feeds could transfer to other chickens and even to humans. The landmark paper concluded that 'These data speak strongly against the unqualified and unlimited use of drug feeds in animal husbandry and speak for revaluation of this form of widespread treatment of animals.'

In 1977, Donald Kennedy who was then the Commissioner of the US FDA attempted to ban antibiotics in agricultural growth promotion. According to a story in the *Washington Post*, 'That effort was quickly halted under pressure from industry groups and pharmaceutical companies, which said there were gaps in the research.'

Just as with environmental pollution, the specific link between antibiotic use in animals and drug-resistant infections in humans is difficult to prove. Despite these challenges, there is substantial evidence suggesting that antibiotic use in agriculture contributes to the rise in antibiotic-resistant superbugs. There are over a hundred studies that provide evidence of the connection between animal antibiotic consumption and antibiotic-resistant superbugs in humans.

In the absence of any meaningful regulatory action, farmers switched from expensive food for animals to low-cost antibiotics, which boosted livestock growth while diminishing production expenses. Predominant food producers institutionalized antibiotics into their production systems, not only to spur growth but also to address ailments in animals. Quite remarkably, after dumping antibiotics into animals and the environment for decades, we still don't know quite why they have growth-enhancing effects. It is possible this has something to do with changes in the bacteria the animals harbour in their microbiomes.

Today, we are caught in a web that has been spun from decades of antibiotic misuse, not only in human medicine but also in animal farming. While doctors overprescribed antibiotics to humans, farmers inundated animals with these drugs, creating a perfect storm for the development and spread of antibiotic-resistant bacteria. In fact, it is estimated that over 70 per cent of antibiotics – including drugs of last resort – are used as cheap food additives to fatten animals meant for consumption.

The implications are frightening, both for public health and food security. Bacteria acquire resistance genes, negating the benefits of antibiotics and rendering them useless in treating infections. But agricultural interests are not incentivized to act against this. Instead of keeping animals in clean enclosures and treating them compassionately, they're fed drugs as growth promoters while being kept in unhygienic conditions.

Unfortunately, the same antibiotics that are prescribed to people are often used for livestock. It seems clear that the movement of bacteria between animals and humans could very well lead to the spread of new resistance genes in superbugs. This shouldn't come as a surprise because, as the COVID-19 pandemic reminded us, humans live in an environment shared with animals. The 'One Health' principle I introduced in the previous chapter recognizes that the health of humans, animals, and the environment is interlinked. This principle advocates for an integrated approach in addressing health challenges, emphasizing collaborative efforts across various disciplines to achieve optimal health outcomes for people, animals, and our shared environment.

We have already discussed one of the major fallouts from ignoring the fact that human health is connected to the health of animals and to the environment. As I mentioned in Chapter 5, in 2015 researchers found a mobile gene in bacteria resistant to the last-resort antibiotic colistin from a pig in China. Shortly thereafter, colistin-resistant superbugs were found in humans.

In 2016, all 193 member states of the United Nations signed an agreement recognizing antibiotic use in agriculture as a driver of antibiotic resistance. Margaret Chan, then Director-General of WHO, emphasized the urgent need for action, saying, 'We are running out of time.' In 2018, a widely published investigative report commissioned by the Bureau of Investigative Journalism found that at least five animal pharmaceutical companies in India unabashedly promoted products containing colistin as growth enhancers. The reporters focused on one company – Venky's – which promoted colistin to Indian farmers. At the time, their product packaging, adorned with cheerful chickens, suggests that it 'improves weight gain'. The reporters were able to purchase 200 grams of Venky's colistin product over the counter in Bengaluru without any prescription. But Venky's was not breaking any laws by selling colistin.

Shortly after the report was published, the Indian government took decisive action by banning the use of colistin in farms. In this instance, the government should be applauded for taking decisive action. But more needs to be done. All antibiotics critical for human health should be banned from agricultural use. Until laws addressing antibiotic resistance and superbugs can be established and effectively enforced, it is essential to have more transparent labelling for animals used for food, indicating whether they were raised with antibiotics. Let informed consumers know which of their meat and dairy products have been raised on antibiotics.

The Indian government's ban on the agricultural use of colistin echoes the lessons learned from diclofenac, a pain relief medication. Once used in cattle, diclofenac led to a drastic decline in South Asia's vulture populations due to its toxicity. Both these cases underline the unintended consequences of using pharmaceuticals in agriculture. While intended to boost productivity and animal health, they can have catastrophic effects on the environment and human health.

12

A Market Failure

The easy availability of antibiotics marked a revolutionary era in healthcare, turning once-fatal infections into mere nuisances. However, as Scott Podolsky highlights, this innovation came at a cost. Dubbed 'the Antibiotics Era', the period following the Second World War saw an explosion in the discovery and commercialization of new antibiotics.

Initially, antibiotics were seen as miracle drugs. Because penicillin, the trailblazer, was not patented, there was a global hunt for new, patentable antibiotics. The pharmaceutical industry responded with zeal, discovering and patenting a slew of antibiotics between 1948 and 1950. These were aggressively marketed and eagerly prescribed by doctors, leading to a surge in usage.

Another big milestone was Selman Waksman's discovery of streptomycin in 1943, and equally important was the method he worked out to systematically search for antibiotics. The Waksman platform was the gold standard for the next two decades. However, like any Gold Rush, this era soon faced its challenges.

The same compounds kept resurfacing when soil samples were screened for antibiotics. Parallel to this was the rise of the synthetic compounds that chemists made in the laboratory. But despite their promise, only the fluoroquinolones emerged as a broad-spectrum class of antibacterial drugs in the 1970s and 1980s. The stumbling block was the bacterial cell envelope which proved to be a daunting fortress.

So, where does this leave us today?

The WHO gathers and reviews information on the pipeline of new treatments targeting bacterial diseases. Their assessment covers antibiotics, synthetic antibacterial drugs, as well as other experimental treatments. The focus lies on the most harmful bacteria, which are termed 'priority pathogens'. While not formally dubbed priority pathogens, the WHO also assesses *Mycobacterium tuberculosis* which causes TB and *Clostridioides difficile*, the bacterium that causes diarrhoea and colitis which we discussed in Chapter 8. In 2022, a WHO report identified forty-six antibiotics and thirty-four non-traditional antibacterial treatments under clinical development as of November 2021.

While this number might seem substantial, in comparison to the drug pipeline for other major diseases such as cancer, there are woefully few drugs in development to treat bacterial infections. WHO highlights that roughly a third of development initiatives are abandoned each year. The reality is that many promising candidates don't reach the market either because they don't work in subsequent trials or due to lack of commercial viability.

Between 2017 and 2021, only twelve new antibacterial drugs received approval. While this number may seem large, only two – vaborbactam combined with meropenem and lefamulin – showed 'distinct modes of action' or belonged to 'unique chemical classes' under the metrics that the WHO uses to gauge innovation. Vaborbactam is notable for its effectiveness against Gram-negative superbugs resistant to carbapenem, whereas lefamulin introduces a new chemical class of drugs. Cefiderocol also stood out as another antibacterial drug effective against Gram-negative superbugs, including carbapenem-resistant *Acinetobacter baumannii* and *Pseudomonas aeruginosa*, though it doesn't strictly fit the WHO's innovation standards.

Regrettably, most other antibiotics and antibacterial drugs approved within this period were derivatives of their predecessors. Given that these drugs were derived from existing antibiotics for which resistant superbugs already exist, the likelihood of resistance to these is also quite high. Considering these hurdles, the current clinical pipeline – with fewer than fifty potential drugs and only a dozen approvals – is simply insufficient to tackle superbugs.

The primary concerns with our current options to treat

bacterial infections are a lack of originality and limited potency against resistant superbugs. Addressing these gaps requires profound strategic rethinking, economic incentives, and genuine innovation. The problem looks even more stark when we consider that bringing a drug from discovery through approval to market can take ten to fifteen years. In that time, tens of millions of people could die from superbug infections. Ideally, we would want new antibacterial drugs to be available before resistance developed to our last lines of defence.

But then what about the headlines that appear from time to time about how a university academic lab researcher has found a promising drug to treat superbugs? Without diminishing the effort and significance of these studies, I think they must be put into context. Even for drugs that show great promise, what needs to be understood is there's a long road ahead. These drugs must undergo testing in clinical trials and statistically a new drug, any drug, has a slim chance of receiving approval.

Researchers often sift through thousands of chemical compounds to find one that might work as an antibiotic. Identifying a promising molecule is just the beginning; it then takes years to perfect it, produce it in large quantities, and confirm that it's safe for humans. Preclinical tests can take over five years, and only a few molecules clear this process.

Clinical trials are even more stringent and expensive. A small number of healthy volunteers first receive the drug in

Phase 1 trials to check for side effects and proper dosing. Only about one-third of drugs pass this phase. In Phase 2, the drug is tested on a small group of patients to see if it's effective. If successful, Phase 3 involves testing on thousands of patients over several years to confirm efficacy and identify any rare side effects.

Following the completion of clinical trials, the drug must receive approval from national regulatory authorities before it can be mass produced and sold. In the US, this regulatory body is the FDA. In India, the equivalent authority is the Central Drugs Standard Control Organization. Only after gaining approval from these regulatory bodies can a new drug enter the market.

There are significant costs to every step of this process of research and development, followed by clearances and finally, mass production. At each stage, companies must critically evaluate a new drug's efficacy and safety to decide whether to proceed further. Some estimates peg the costs of getting through Phase 3 of trials as billions of dollars. What's more, this cost doesn't even account for regulatory requirements, susceptibility testing, and manufacturing. To give you an idea of the manufacturing complexity, sourcing raw materials for an antibiotic can take up to eight months, and the actual manufacturing process can add an additional fourteen months.

And even after approvals, drugs may not perform as well on the market as expected, and they can be withdrawn due to safety concerns arising post approval or simply due to poor sales. To make matters worse, antibiotics have the highest withdrawal rate of any class of medicine. Any pharmaceutical company would naturally want to recoup the costs of their research and development efforts and make a profit. Rationally, when you bring a product to market, you want to sell as many units of it as you can at the highest possible price. But this business model runs contrary to the key characteristics of antibiotics that make them unfavourable for generating huge profits.

Antibiotics usually have lower prices than other types of drugs, and depending on the country, companies are granted a monopoly on their products for about twenty years. However, much of this time is consumed by clinical trials, leaving them roughly ten years to make profits and recoup costs. At the end of this period, the drug's value plummets as it is no longer patented and generic versions emerge.

Substitutes then become easily available, reducing the incentives to invest in new antibiotics. A generic version of a drug costs much less since the research and development costs have been absorbed by the company that brought it to market first. Doctors and patients will typically use a less expensive generic antibiotic if it effectively treats an infection, further reducing the need for newer, patented drugs. This preference for generics means that the market for patented antibiotics is considerably smaller than for generics. Since affordable alternatives are readily available, patented

A Market Failure

antibiotics only account for a small fraction of sales in the market. Thus, when generic drugs dominate the market, pharmaceutical companies lack the financial incentive to invest in new antibiotic research and development.

There's also a disconnect between an antibiotic's societal value and the price it commands in the market. Patient awareness is also often lacking, as they do not always understand the true value of advanced antibiotic treatments. Typically, an antibiotic is prescribed for only a short course, often just a few days. That's because if an antibiotic works well, the infection clears up rapidly. This contrasts with the medicines used to keep chronic conditions like statins that regulate cholesterol or, for example, the new blockbuster class of glucagon-like peptide 1 (GLP-1) drugs that reduce obesity. Those are long-term generators of revenue for pharmaceutical companies. The short-term use of antibiotics limits the revenue a pharmaceutical company can earn from each prescription, making the market less appealing for potential investors.

New antibiotics are also a precious resource, something that should be used as a last resort. They are intentionally held in reserve to prevent overuse and the spread of bacterial resistance. As we know, there is also the ticking clock of developing bacterial resistance in the background. Once that happens, an antibiotic can be rendered ineffective even before it has recouped development costs, creating further difficulty in the pricing structure.

Experts agree that due to these reasons, the economic incentives to produce new antibiotics are distorted and therefore, we can't simply rely on market forces to produce new antibiotics. However, given the issue of increasing bacterial resistance, the need to find new drugs is becoming more urgent. Some suggestions for this include redesigning clinical trials for broader participation, especially in countries where drug-resistant infections are common. Another idea is to have more focused incentive programmes that support drug development at every stage. But regardless of the approach, the goal remains the same: we must find ways to encourage the development of essential new drugs.

Developing new drugs is a complex and costly process. Recognizing this, governments and global organizations have been trying to incentivize the discovery of new antibiotics, through various schemes that offer rewards and support. These come in two forms: push incentives, which help lower research and development costs, and pull incentives, which are designed to help these drugs successfully enter the market.

Push incentives support the early and riskiest phases of drug development, and they aim to reduce the costs and challenges associated with it. They make vital research tools available, invest in scientific training, and provide direct research funding. In essence, push incentives not only offer financial support but also create an environment that fosters drug development. They form a critical foundation in addressing the unpredictability of antimicrobial resistance and preparing us for the health challenges of the future.

Successful examples of these schemes include the Community for Open Antimicrobial Drug Discovery, which uses advanced methods to test potential drugs against five of the Deadly Six superbugs and two disease-causing fungi. This service, which is free to researchers worldwide, has examined over 300,000 compounds from over 43 countries. Other efforts involve making data about resistant organisms available to researchers and funding foundational research that helps us understand the interaction between hosts and pathogens.

Further, push incentives also play a crucial role in the middle stages of drug development. Various institutions and collaborations offer funding and support for preclinical research and early clinical trials. One example is CARB-X, or Combating Antibiotic-Resistant Bacteria Biopharmaceutical Accelerator, a global non-profit which focuses on priority pathogens and provides funding for the riskiest stages of product development. Not only does CARB-X focus on antibiotics, but it also supports projects for other drugs, vaccines, and diagnostics. From 2016 to 2022, CARB-X propelled eighteen projects into or through human clinical trials. Of these, two were launched on the market and seven had secured partnerships for further development.

Global collaboration is another important aspect of many of these incentives. Partnerships like the Global Antibiotic

Research and Development Partnership work on developing new antibacterial medicines and ensuring access in countries where they are most needed. This partnership was established through a collaboration between the WHO and the Drugs for Neglected Diseases initiative. It has the ambitious goal of delivering five new treatments by 2025.

On the flip side, pull incentives try to guarantee market success for new drugs. These can be either direct financial rewards or benefits like faster regulatory reviews or extended market exclusivity. Making new drugs available and affordable is a huge challenge. Even when financial help is available, new medicines are still often more expensive than older, generic ones. This means that even though there's a need for new treatments, they aren't always used as much as they should be.

Different countries have adopted different approaches. In France and Germany, antibiotic reimbursement programmes are being implemented with a focus on establishing minimum price guarantees. This is designed to ensure that antibiotics remain financially viable for manufacturers and addresses the challenge of developing new antibiotics under traditional market conditions. By guaranteeing a minimum price, these programmes provide a more predictable and sustainable revenue model for antibiotic developers.

It is a known fact that India's pharmaceutical market is highly competitive and price sensitive. Implementing a minimum price guarantee model for antibiotics in a country like India, which has an uneven healthcare system comprising a mix of public and private sectors, is challenging. The public healthcare system often struggles with underfunding and limited resources, making it difficult to institute broad, government-backed pricing guarantees.

However, sometimes, incentives end up promoting small tweaks to existing drugs rather than promoting groundbreaking new ones. This happens because minor modifications often bring quicker returns, making them more attractive to companies.

In the US, while there are several pull incentives in place, their effectiveness is debatable. Challenges in the system mean that certain schemes might not have the desired impact. Specifically, reward systems intended to motivate hospitals to adopt new drugs frequently become entangled in bureaucratic complexities. This red tape can obscure the effectiveness of the incentives, making it difficult to determine if they are truly encouraging the adoption and use of new medical treatments as intended. In essence, the pull system's effectiveness is compromised by administrative hurdles, rather than the efficacy of the drugs being questioned.

To encourage companies to make new antibiotics, there have been some suggestions about providing a special financial reward once a new antibiotic is approved. This idea has gained a lot of attention. However, there's a great deal of debate about how much this reward should be or how such incentives could be structured. Some experts suggest rewards could range from US$500 million to $1billion for each new antibiotic. The UK has proposed paying companies over US$140 million for each new antibiotic they develop. There's even been talk of a combined effort from the world's twenty largest economies to offer US$4 billion for every new antibiotic. Incentive structures could involve upfront payments, market entry rewards or long-term contracts to purchase the antibiotics.

Overall, more needs to be done to ensure that a steady stream of new antibiotics is being developed. Today, antibiotic prices as set by market forces don't consider the broader value that these vital life-saving drugs have for society nor do they consider the rise of superbugs.

The development of daptomycin, the last truly innovative class of antibiotic discovered, illustrates the lengthy and complex process of bringing a new drug to market. Discovered in 1984, daptomycin's journey to FDA approval in 2003 spanned nearly two decades. Initial work on daptomycin began in the late 1980s at Eli Lilly and Company, driven by the emergence of bacteria resistant to existing antibiotics like vancomycin. However, early clinical studies revealed that the drug led to muscle toxicity, leading Eli Lilly to discontinue its development in the early 1990s. The project was later revived by Cubist Pharmaceuticals, who licensed daptomycin from Eli Lilly. Overcoming toxicity concerns, Cubist successfully developed the drug for clinical use.

The development of daptomycin is a testament to the

A Market Failure

perseverance and innovation needed in antibiotic research and development, especially given the current drought in discovering new antibiotic classes and the growing threat of superbugs.

But we must remember that even when vital antibiotics work, they're not guaranteed to succeed. Commercialization is often the hardest hurdle. A news article in the *Wall Street Journal* published in September 2023 with the title 'The World Needs New Antibiotics. The Problem Is, No One Can Make Them Profitably' summed up this plight in the first paragraph:

> Six start-ups have won Food and Drug Administration approval for new antibiotics since 2017. All have filed for bankruptcy, been acquired or are shutting down. About 80% of the 300 scientists who worked at the companies have abandoned antibiotic development according to Kevin Outterson, executive director of CARB-X, a government-funded group promoting research in the field.

Two other examples, which serve as cautionary tales, are worth sharing.

Carbapenem-resistant bacteria include Deadly Six superbugs like *E. coli* and *Klebsiella pneumoniae*, and they're recognized as priority pathogens by the WHO. When the FDA approved plazomicin, a new drug targeting these superbugs, in 2018, there was a lot of hope and projections of huge sales. Despite these expectations and the WHO rapidly listing plazomicin as an essential medicine, the drug's sales fell flat, earning only about US$1 million in its first year compared to the projected US$500 million. As a matter of reference, the total sales of all branded antibiotics in 2018 were US$535 million.

Achaogen, the company behind plazomicin, had received substantial funding, including over US$136 million from the Biomedical Advanced Research and Development Authority, US$80 million from various US agencies, and contributions from the Wellcome Trust. Yet, Achaogen faced financial decline around the drug's launch, a common challenge in the antibiotic industry, leading to bankruptcy in 2019. One key issue was that plazomicin was approved only for complicated urinary tract infections, not a broader range of superbug infections, due to challenges in recruiting enough participants for its clinical trial.

Plazomicin's journey is a textbook case highlighting the mismatch between the need for new antibiotics and their success in the marketplace. This situation has sparked calls for rethinking how clinical trials are designed and conducted, with a specific focus on advocating for more global participation to ensure these vital drugs reach the regions where they are most needed.

Nabriva Therapeutics, which developed the antibacterial drug lefamulin for the treatment of community-acquired pneumonia in adults, struggled to achieve commercial success after they launched. A significant factor contributing to Nabriva's struggles was the pricing of lefamulin. The company set the cost for a five-day treatment course at over US$1,000 (₹83,000 at the time of writing). This pricing was substantially higher compared to the generic antibiotics commonly used to treat pneumonia outside of hospital settings. This stark price difference played a crucial role in the market's response to the drug.

Market dynamics and pricing strategies eventually posed significant barriers to lefamulin's broader acceptance and use in the treatment of pneumonia, ultimately impacting Nabriva's operations and sustainability. In 2023, four years after FDA approval, it had to let go of its sixty remaining employees.

The paradox of drug pricing and the challenge it presents is summed up aptly in *Superbugs: An Arms Race against Bacteria* by William Hall, Anthony McDonnell and Jim O'Neill:

> Insurers and governments are willing to pay hundreds of thousands of dollars for a cancer treatment to extend life for just a couple of months, yet they are willing to pay only a fraction of that amount for antibiotics that would cure a patient completely.

Despite all these challenges, there is still hope. India with its vast pharmaceutical industry, large and diverse population, and educated workforce can take a leadership role in developing the next generation of antibacterial drugs from discovery to clinical trials to approval. This can also be done at a fraction of the cost of drug development in Western countries. Public and private partnerships can ensure that incentives are in place and risks are mitigated.

Getting a drug to market when there is a health crisis doesn't have to take a decade or longer, either. We learned this from the COVID-19 pandemic when safe and effective vaccines were developed in under a year, and the first made-for-purpose COVID-19 antiviral drugs received full approval in under two years.

Identifying new antibacterial drugs is possible if, as a society, we recognize the damage caused by superbugs and prioritize tackling the infections they cause. By investing in research and harnessing our collective ingenuity, we can unlock new discoveries. History shows that when humanity unites for a common goal, breakthroughs are achieved.

13

The Next Generation

As we grapple with the looming crisis of antibiotic resistance, an important question must be answered: where will we find the next generation of antibacterial drugs?

In this chapter, I want to highlight some of the most exciting new work on finding new antibiotics, creating antibacterial drugs chemically, and using new tools such as artificial intelligence (AI) to test for antibacterial properties. All of these approaches are in the early stages and might not make it through the gauntlet of animal and human clinical trials. But they give us a flavour of the innovation involved (often from laboratories in academic institutions and start-ups) in identifying promising leads.

So, where might new antibiotics come from? One promising avenue is to return to the soil, where antibiotics were originally discovered. The earth beneath our feet teems with microbes that have spent billions of years in an arms race competing for resources, resulting in the natural development of antibiotic substances.

The significance of soil-dwelling bacteria in antibiotic discovery cannot be overstated. During the early days of antibiotic discovery, perhaps 80 per cent of all antibiotics were derived from a single kind of bacteria, *Streptomyces*. Many of these soil bacteria gave rise to many of the other kinds of drugs in use today.

The systematic approach spearheaded by soil microbiologist Selman Waksman screened cultivable soil microbes to isolate antibiotics such as streptomycin. However, by the 1960s, this pool of easily accessible antibiotics had largely been tapped out. And when chemists got better at making molecules, scientists in the pharmaceutical industry thought they could get ahead of nature in making antibacterial compounds themselves. But they soon found that these artificial compounds couldn't replace the richness of the natural products isolated from microbes. You see, evolution is a much more elegant chemist than us!

At this juncture, I want to take a detour to describe just how vital soil bacteria have been to medicine by focusing on just one species – *Streptomyces rapamycinicus*. This microbe isolated from soil samples from Easter Island (also known as Rapa Nui) has given the world many drugs. These include hygromycin, an antibiotic, and rapamycin, an antifungal drug that also serves as an immunosuppressant in organ transplantation.

The Next Generation

Easter Island, while famed for its iconic Moai statues, caught the attention of microbiologist Georges Nógrády for a completely different reason. In 1964, Nógrády observed that the barefoot inhabitants of Easter Island weren't afflicted by tetanus, a surprising fact given the abundance of horses, which are a common source of this bacterial disease. He collected various soil samples, hoping to find a chemical answer. Although he didn't find the tetanus spores he sought, he passed the samples to Ayerst Pharmaceuticals (modern-day Pfizer), where scientists were in pursuit of medical compounds produced by bacteria.

In a rather serendipitous turn of events, the Ayerst team identified a novel antifungal drug which they christened rapamycin in honour of the Polynesian name of the island. While rapamycin is ineffective against bacteria, it is especially effective against disease-causing fungi.

But the story doesn't end here. The world owes the continued existence of rapamycin in great part to Surendra Nath Sehgal, a microbiologist of Indian origin. Many years later, after research on rapamycin was abandoned, Sehgal was instrumental in saving samples, even maintaining many in the freezer of his refrigerator at home.

Born in 1932 in a small village in what is now part of Pakistan, Sehgal obtained both a bachelor's and master's degree in pharmacy from Banaras Hindu University. This was followed by research at Bristol University in the UK. Sehgal's doctoral thesis focused on the impact of antibiotics on microorganisms, specifically the action of streptomycin on *Staphylococcus aureus*.

When Ayerst Laboratories decided to close their lab in Montreal in 1983 and discard all non-viable compounds, Sehgal took a defiant and history-altering step. His side experiments, including an effective, albeit likely illegal treatment for a neighbour's fungal infection, showcased its potential. Instead of destroying rapamycin, he took a few glass vials of the bacteria and kept them in his freezer with a note cautioning, 'DON'T EAT!'

Sehgal's journey with rapamycin continued in New Jersey with Ayerst, and later with Wyeth, the new owners of the company. Soon, it became evident that the compound had another valuable trait – it could suppress the immune system. Under Sehgal's guidance, this compound was eventually transformed into a clinically recognized medication that prevents organ transplant rejection. It is also used in treating certain types of cancer.

But we don't have to restrict ourselves to soil to find new antibiotics. Recent research has shown that diverse and previously unexplored environments, including oceans and even the nests of fungus-farming ants, could also be valuable sources of new antibiotics. Astonishingly, 99 per cent of all microbial species in external environments like the soil and oceans are 'uncultured', meaning they do not readily grow under laboratory conditions. This vast biological wilderness is largely unexplored but highly promising.

The Next Generation

In recent years, researchers have developed new techniques to tap into this untamed reservoir. By cultivating these bacteria in their natural environments or using specific growth factors, scientists have managed to bring these elusive organisms into laboratory settings for study. The results have been promising so far. Compounds like lassomycin, and other natural products from marine sponges, indicate that uncultured organisms hold a treasure trove of antimicrobial potential. Unlike their cultured counterparts, uncultured bacteria might provide us with antibiotics with new modes of action, dramatically expanding the possibilities for drug development.

Scientists have also made a remarkable discovery regarding other bacteria that are hard to grow in laboratories. They found a new antibiotic called teixobactin using a unique method that allows these bacteria to grow in specially designed chambers. Teixobactin is an exceptional antibiotic that doesn't target usual bacterial defences, making it hard for bacteria to develop resistance to it. It targets a vulnerable part of harmful bacteria, specifically in a component used to build their protective walls. Thus, it can effectively kill or stop the growth of these harmful bacteria. In addition, it works through a two-step process so resistant bacteria need to defeat both steps to overcome the antibiotic. It's part of a new group of antibiotics and has shown promise in fighting drug-resistant diseases when tested on animals.

The next key step will be to see if the promise of teixobactin holds up in human trials. And as we discussed in Chapter 12, even if it does, it may be years before the antibiotic is in the market. Still, the discovery of teixobactin from previously uncultured bacteria offers a glimmer of hope. It not only emphasizes that nature still hides potent tools for medicine, but it also hints at a renaissance in discovering drugs from natural sources.

These are examples of antibiotics isolated from microbes. But chemists can also help with creating new antibacterial compounds. Given the significant expertise in chemistry due to a large technically skilled base of researchers, India can play a major role and become a powerhouse in drug design and discovery.

India is already the world's largest producer of vaccines and generic medicines with further growth expected. While it is useful to produce generics at scale, innovation in medicines will become increasingly crucial, especially with respect to new patentable drugs like antibacterials. Collaborations between the government and industry have been a key factor in strengthening India's position in the global pharmaceutical market. The transition to innovation will be accelerated by increasing research and development investments, an emphasis on robust intellectual property laws, and rights and efforts to harmonize regulatory requirements to global standards.

As we discussed in Chapter 12, pharmaceutical giants are reluctant to develop new antibiotics since they're expensive to produce and don't promise high returns. Anand Kumar, co-founder of Bugworks Research, a small company based in Bengaluru, aims to address this gap. Having switched from designing computer chips to drug discovery after his recovery from cancer, Anand has a personal motivation to succeed – he lost his father to an antibiotic-resistant superbug.

Under the direction of chemist Shahul Hameed, Bugworks has created a compound they call BWC0977, which seems to be effective against superbugs that are resistant to many existing antibiotics, including fluoroquinolones, carbapenems, and colistin. The team created fewer than a hundred chemical compounds based on the shapes of the business ends of the target enzymes.

BWC0977 targets two key bacterial enzymes that are crucial for bacterial survival and spread. Hitting two targets reduces the chances of resistance developing. It is difficult to predict whether the compound will work and whether it will receive the financial backing for successful commercialization, but we need more companies like Bugworks to take the initiative in antibacterial drug discovery. At the time of writing, BWC0977 had progressed to early-stage clinical trials to determine safety for human use.

Chemists are also finding new ways to create antibiotics that look and behave like natural ones. The antibiotic erythromycin, first isolated in 1952 from a soil sample from the Philippines, has been a mainstay in treating bacterial infections. However, its natural form is far from ideal. It is unstable in the acidic environment of the stomach and can even transform into a toxic compound. Over the years, chemists have tweaked erythromycin to improve its stability and reduce toxicity. Yet, as antibiotic-resistant bacteria emerged, the options for modifying this complex molecule have dwindled.

Chemist Andrew Myers and his team at Harvard University decided to tackle this challenge by synthesizing erythromycin variations from scratch. Myers and his team have come up with an exciting new way to create antibiotics. Instead of traditional stepwise chemical methods, they use a set of eight easily available chemicals to create building blocks. By assembling them in various ways, they can form new ring-shaped compounds. So far, they've made over 350 of these compounds, and many of these seem to work like natural antibiotics. What's exciting is that two of these antibiotics are effective against drug-resistant superbugs in laboratory settings.

Of course, developing potential new antibiotics in the lab is just the first step. But there's a silver lining. Myers' method is more direct and straightforward than the old ways of tweaking existing antibiotics. So, even if the road ahead is long, this new approach might lead to other powerful antibiotics in the future.

Another cutting-edge approach is protein engineering. By understanding how the proteins involved in creating antibiotics work, it might be possible to edit them to produce new forms of antibiotics. This would represent a significant advancement in creating variations of antibiotics that keep us one step ahead of superbugs.

Scientists are also using approaches that merge newer technologies like genetic engineering, protein engineering, and synthetic biology with standard microbiology and chemistry. For instance, it's possible to genetically modify bacteria, making them conducive to manipulation, and transform them into antibiotic production units by introducing potential antibiotic genes identified from the environment. This approach could also lead to the identification of 'hidden antibiotics' if we can perfectly replicate the conditions in which these antibiotics are made naturally.

Some scientists are taking yet another approach. Can AI help find antibacterial drugs that beat superbugs? Since the launch of large language models in 2022, there's been rapid interest in using AI in various applications. But AI isn't simply confined to chatbots that generate text and images. There's much interest in using AI to discover new drugs.

So, how exactly does AI help? Since the chemical universe is incredibly large, AI filters out promising compounds for specific diseases in a faster and cheaper manner. In principle, AI could also come up with drugs that humans wouldn't think of rationally. One of the superpowers of AI is that the path to discovery doesn't need to be charted specifically by humans to the AI model. It's a case where the black-box intelligence of AI might come in handy.

Today, researchers are working on next-generation compounds that act more like snipers than carpet bombers. These compounds aim to target specific bacteria, sparing the beneficial microbes that make up our microbiome. By doing so, they hope to minimize collateral damage and reduce the selective pressures leading to the evolution of resistance, and AI can be used to identify these compounds.

For example, led by American biological engineer James Collins, researchers from the Massachusetts Institute of Technology and McMaster University are using deep learning, a kind of AI approach that teaches computers to handle data like the human brain, to identify promising chemical compounds for testing as superbug-killers. Reporting their work in scientific journals, these researchers have identified likely compounds, including two which they've named halicin and abaucin. In laboratory settings, these have been shown to thwart specific superbugs. What's more, the approach that the team used could also be helpful in finding promising drug candidates for other diseases.

In a paper published in *Nature Chemical Biology* in May 2023, the researchers focused on one of our Deadly Six superbugs, *Acinetobacter baumannii*. The compound they identified, abaucin, is highly potent against this superbug and has limited effect on other bacteria. This is a desirable trait in an antibacterial drug since broad-spectrum antibiotics can indiscriminately kill both good and bad bacteria. Earlier, in 2020, the same researchers had shown the effectiveness of

The Next Generation

the AI approach in identifying halicin, an antibiotic effective against multiple superbugs. In that case, the AI model had been trained to find drugs that stopped the growth of *E. coli*.

In December 2023, as I was finishing up writing this book, Collins's team reported using AI that not only predicts whether a compound will be a good antibiotic but also explains which parts of its structure make it effective. This is a big step forward because it helps us understand what makes an antibiotic work at a deeper, structural level. One of the new types of compounds they discovered is especially effective against superbugs like MRSA and vancomycin-resistant bacteria.

Armed with these successes, the team plans to extend their AI-based approach to find candidate antibiotics that fight infection caused by other superbugs. The results are quite encouraging.

What's more, finding new drugs isn't the only way AI might help defeat superbugs. AI could support us in optimizing existing antibiotics and help doctors diagnose and treat infections with our existing arsenal of antibiotics. At present, it's hard to say with any certainty that the AI models in use now will lead to the next life-saving antibacterial drugs. But I think these early steps are promising. AI will get faster and better, and given the scale of the problem of superbugs, we will need all the help we can get.

Predicting which research approaches will lead to the discovery of new antibiotics and antibacterial treatments is difficult. But by diversifying efforts – much like increasing the number of arrows launched towards a target – we increase the chance of hitting the bullseye.

Traditional drugs aren't the only way to treat superbug infections either. There are other avenues for treatment that also hold promise and merit our attention. Let's look into a few of these.

14

Beyond Antibiotics

Phages

Tom Patterson and Steffanie Strathdee never expected a normal vacation to take such a scary turn. The couple were both scientists at the University of California in San Diego, and they had embarked on a trip to Egypt. And as they had hoped, the journey was incredible. Their final destination was the Valley of the Kings, and they reached it by taking an overnight boat trip on the Nile. The couple enjoyed a peaceful evening on the deck of the ship. However, the serenity was short-lived. Once they returned to their cabin, Patterson began to feel ill, vomiting repeatedly. Initially, they thought it was just a bout of food poisoning.

Later the pair would discover that Patterson was suffering from an infection with a life-threatening superbug, one of our Deadly Six, *Acinetobacter baumannii*. The superbug was resistant to eighteen antibiotics, including the last resort drug colistin (which we covered in Chapter 5). Only through an incredible confluence of events and Strathdee's research into a treatment option that had fallen out of favour in Western medical practice would her husband's life be saved. She later recounted the entire ordeal in her book, *The Perfect Predator*.

The outline of the story is worth telling here. After the initial discovery in Egypt, Patterson was airlifted to Frankfurt due to the severity of his condition. Here, doctors discovered a football-sized abscess in his gut. His condition continued to deteriorate, and he fell into a medically induced coma. Patterson was then transferred back to San Diego. The superbug seemed unbeatable, showing resistance to even the few remaining antibiotics. Doctors faced an immediate dilemma on how to treat the abscess. They could perform surgery or attempt to drain the infected fluid. If the infection entered his bloodstream, Patterson could suffer from septic shock. In such a state, the body signals a frantic red alert, causing the blood pressure to plummet, heart rate to surge, and the breathing to quicken. This condition can escalate swiftly, carrying a 50 per cent chance of death. Given these stakes, the medical team decided against surgery, choosing instead to insert five drains into Tom's abdomen to remove the fluid.

Unfortunately, Patterson's health took a hit when one of his abdominal drains slipped, causing him to go into septic shock. He was quickly taken back to the ICU and placed on a ventilator for breathing support.

As Patterson was on the verge of death, Strathdee, who, by extraordinary luck happened to be an infectious disease epidemiologist, researched a last-resort solution online: bacteriophage therapy. This was a century-old treatment that used viruses called bacteriophages (or phages for short) to kill bacteria. Though no longer commonly used after the advent of antibiotics, Strathdee remembered reading about phages and decided to explore this avenue.

Strathdee gained approval for experimental treatment under humanitarian grounds from the FDA and started an international search for compatible phages, turning her quest into a global endeavour involving researchers from around the world.

Speaking later to the BBC, Strathdee recalled the episode: 'We essentially had phage researchers from all over the world who were offering help – from Switzerland, Belgium, Poland, the Republic of Georgia, India. The Belgians even offered for their phage to be sent in a diplomatic pouch. These were total strangers who had stepped up to the plate, a true global village to rescue one man.'

Within three weeks, a cocktail of four phages was ready for Patterson, who was now on full life support. Strathdee knew that she was taking a huge risk with experimental therapy, but doing nothing wasn't an option. The first phage cocktail was injected into Patterson's abdomen, followed later by a more potent cocktail administered intravenously. Astonishingly, he woke up from his coma three days later. Despite additional bouts of septic shock and complications, Patterson eventually recovered, making him the first person in North America to receive intravenous phage therapy for a superbug infection throughout the body.

Strathdee had utilized her own scientific background and a global network of researchers to find a solution, and Patterson fought on, even when he was at the edge of death. 'As an infectious disease epidemiologist, having my husband dying from a superbug was just a shock,' Strathdee later said. The event turned Strathdee into an advocate for phage therapy, and she began receiving calls from people worldwide looking for a way to combat superbug infections afflicting their loved ones.

A year into Patterson's recovery, his case was showcased at the Institut Pasteur in Paris during a meeting commemorating the hundredth anniversary of the discovery of the bacteriophage, the biological entity that had saved his life – a happy ending if ever there was one.

Today, as we grapple with the limitations of antibiotics, phages are making a comeback. So let's dive into phages: what are they and why were they forgotten?

Phages are viruses that infect and kill specific bacterial cells. They are the ultimate bacterial predators, making up the most numerous biological entities on Earth. They are everywhere in the environment – the air, water, soil, and even inside us right now. Scientists think there are around 10 trillion viruses inside each of us, and most of them are phages that hunt bacteria! We have not identified most of them, but what's almost certain is that they influence our microbiomes and our health in ways that we have yet to discover.

Phages are microscopic marvels to behold. A single phage looks like a tiny lunar lander with a head that holds genetic material and legs that allow it to latch on to bacteria.

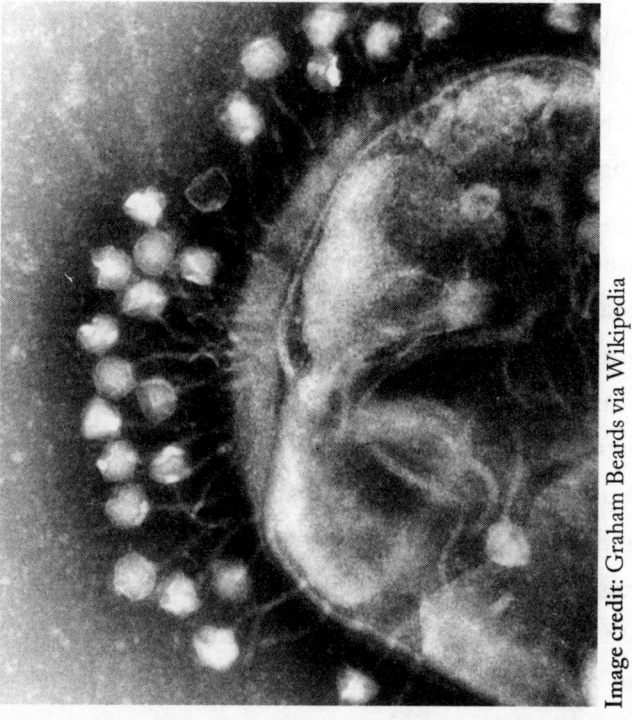

Bacteriophages attacking a bacterial cell at 200,000x magnification, showcasing the intricate interaction between viruses and bacteria.

These microscopic entities may sound terrifying, but they have an incredibly targeted mode of action. A phage latches on to a bacterial cell, injects its DNA, and then commandeers the cell to produce more phages. Eventually, the bacterial cell bursts open, releasing these newly minted phages to continue their battle against bacteria. Unlike antibiotics, which can indiscriminately kill both harmful and beneficial bacteria, phages are highly specific and leave other microbes untouched.

However, not all phages act in this way. Some, known as lysogenic phages, opt for a more temperate life. Instead of causing an explosion, they merge their genes with the bacteria they infect and just lie low. Because they don't kill the bacteria they infect, they can sometimes pick up pieces of bacterial genes. Due to their potential to transfer genes between bacteria, including those responsible for antibiotic resistance, these are not favoured in phage therapy. These viruses can actually make bacteria more resistant to antibiotics and increase their ability to cause harm. To treat bacterial infections, the kind of phages that are most important are the 'tailed' lytic phages, which burst the bacteria they parasitize. This direct and aggressive approach to destroying bacteria makes lytic phages powerful allies against bacterial infections. These also have a low risk of horizontal gene transfer, making them a more controlled and predictable option for treating bacterial infections.

I remember futuristic illustrations of the life cycles of

phages from biology classes in college. But they're not as obscure or recently discovered as they're made out to be. If you or your child studied biology in high school, you may remember their distinctive shape from the biology textbook. In fact, an illustration of a phage features prominently in NCERT textbooks used by Indian schools.

Phage therapy is not new either. In fact, the idea to use phages to kill harmful bacteria goes back to the early twentieth century. The term 'bacteriophage' itself was coined by Canadian microbiologist Felix d'Herelle in 1916, and he used his knowledge to treat soldiers affected by dysentery in the First World War. He and Frederick Twort, who stumbled upon phages from a different research path, are known as the pioneers in understanding these unique viruses.

In the decades that followed, phage research became a prominent scientific endeavour in Georgia, USSR, with most of the work being done at the Eliava Institute in the capital Tbilisi. But with the discovery of antibiotics, phage therapy was largely forgotten in Western countries. Soon, the idea of using phages to treat infections was met with scepticism by most physicians.

Physicians who used phages didn't keep detailed records, and some patients got better on their own or were also taking antibiotics. As a result, no one was quite sure if it was the phage treatment, the body's natural healing, or the antibiotics that did the trick. Hence, the use of phage therapy dwindled, especially when antibiotics, which were much simpler to use, came on the scene.

While this was the situation in most parts of the world, some of the countries of the former Soviet Union continued to use phages. For example, in Georgia, which is a leader in the medical use of phages, they have been in use for decades. You can go to a pharmacy and pick up a vial of phages for common ailments.

Today, phage therapy remains largely underutilized in most countries due to regulatory hurdles and a lack of clinical trials. On the other hand, the use of killer phages is a source of great promise and genuine excitement. First off, they are very selective in what they eat and only target specific bacteria, which means they do not harm the friendly bacteria of the microbiome. Also, when they are introduced to the site of an infection, they replicate easily, increasing their numbers greatly.

These biological alternatives have an evolutionary edge too. Unlike chemical drugs, phages can adapt along with their bacterial targets. Each phage is specific to a type or even a strain of bacteria, requiring careful matching for effective treatment.

To understand the full story of phages, we must travel back to 1896 to India. A brilliant English chemist, Ernest Hankin made a startling discovery while testing the waters of the Ganga and Yamuna rivers. Cholera is endemic in India, and there were several cholera pandemics in the country during the 1800s. Hankin observed that people who lived by many of India's rivers were not prone to the disease. Since cholera is primarily a waterborne disease, he collected samples from rivers. Hankin made the startling discovery that the waters of the Ganga and Yamuna rivers had something in them that could kill *Vibrio cholerae*, the bacterium responsible for cholera.

This led to the obvious question: was there a natural combatant in the water capable of wiping out disease-causing bacteria? Very soon, the defensive ability of the water from the Ganga and the Yamuna was attributed to the action of phages. Let's not forget that this discovery preceded the discovery of antibiotics. It also preceded the official discovery of phages by around two decades. Not everyone is convinced that the bactericidal activity Hankin observed was phages in action, but there are still no other theories that can explain the activity of the river water.

Now, let's return to the present. In a time when the threat of antibiotic resistance looms large, phage therapy stands as a significant, rapidly evolving field that could well become a mainstay of infectious disease treatment. Its versatility, ranging from natural to genetically engineered phages and from one-size-fits-all to highly personalized approaches, makes it an incredibly adaptable and potent weapon in our medical arsenal.

One of the appealing features of phages is their specificity. However, this also means that each phage is effective against only a limited range of bacterial species. This poses challenges for treatment in the absence of exact knowledge about the infectious agent. In the world of antibiotics, you can administer a broad-spectrum antibiotic to cover multiple potential culprits. In contrast, the narrow scope of phage therapy requires the identification of the bacterial species causing the infection, which can be time-consuming.

The answer to the specificity dilemma might lie in phage cocktails or mixtures of different phages with varying host ranges. These can offer an immediate, although still targeted, approach to treating bacterial infections. They allow for the treatment of a bacterial species that has not been identified, and even target a specific type of infection. For example, countries in the former Soviet Union have used 'pyophage' cocktails for infections caused by wounds and 'intestiphage' cocktails for gastrointestinal issues.

But the development of these cocktails is not as simple as mixing phages existing in the wild. The solution might lie in genetic engineering or phage training, a form of artificial evolution where phages are encouraged to adapt to different bacterial hosts. This allows scientists to custom design phages that can target specific bacterial strains or even modify existing ones to broaden their host range. However, the same evolutionary principles that have led to antibiotic-resistant bacteria can also apply to phage therapy. Bacteria can evolve to resist phage attacks through mutations, or by acquiring resistance genes.

Perhaps the greatest limitation to phage therapy is the lack of clinical trials showing their effectiveness. The gold standard in drug research is the large randomized controlled trial where the effects of the drug are compared to a placebo. These are essential for establishing the safety and effectiveness of phage therapy, although they are costly, limited in scope, and have produced mixed results so far.

Right now, there's also the more precarious route of compassionate use, generally sought as a last resort in cases such as Tom Patterson's when antibiotics have failed. This approach poses challenges in establishing proof of efficacy since controls are hard to set and standard antibiotics are often used in combination with phages.

Phage therapy has the potential to change how we deal with bacterial infections, especially as more and more bacteria become resistant to traditional antibiotics. But before it can become a widespread solution, there are many hurdles to overcome. Proper clinical trials are needed to demonstrate the broader applicability of phage therapy.

Clinical reports have significantly increased, from only two in 2015 to around twenty each in 2021 and 2022. Most of these studies are case reports or series that are categorized as compassionate treatments. They do not have control populations, but they provide valuable information on the safety of phage therapy. Even in populations of critically ill patients with conditions like severe sepsis and septic shock, phage therapy has demonstrated safety and efficacy. These studies support the anti-infection effectiveness of phage therapy despite all the acknowledged limitations.

Importantly, phages are a part of the normal human microbiome, especially in the gastrointestinal tract, indicating that they are generally well tolerated by the immune system. Indeed, clinical observations have shown that phage treatments usually result in minimal adverse effects.

There is also an economic challenge to overcome in the research and development of phage therapy. Unlike new drugs made in labs, phages are natural. In places like the US, it's hard to get a patent for biological entities, without which companies are less likely to invest in research. Why spend all that money if someone else can easily copy your discovery?

Genetically engineered phages, with their enhanced antibacterial activity, may offer a workaround for patent issues since these can be patented more easily. Although Western Europe is trying to simplify the rules around phage therapy, the overall rigid approach is holding back its wider use.

Unlike antibiotics, we don't know a lot about how phages move and behave within our bodies. The usual measurements used for drugs, like how much is needed for it to work or how long it stays in the system, aren't clearly established for them. This is partly because unlike regular drugs, they multiply during treatment, making them harder to study.

Another interesting feature of phages is that they can either enhance or reduce the effects of antibiotics. Their effectiveness can change depending on many factors, like the stage of the bacterial infection or the condition of the bacterial cells. Even though they can naturally increase in number when treating an infection, this feature complicates their approval for general use. Given that there are countless varieties of phages, making standard treatment plans is an enormous challenge.

Phage therapy could be particularly promising when conventional treatments have failed, offering a possible lifeline for chronic or drug-resistant infections. For those grappling with antibiotic-resistant infections, phage therapy offers a glimmer of hope. As bacteria continue to outsmart the drugs designed to kill them, it's increasingly clear that a broader arsenal is needed in the fight against superbugs.

It is clear that phage therapy cannot replace antibiotics because phages are not a scalable option to deal with the magnitude of the superbug crisis. However, it is possible that they could serve as an additional tool to fight against resistant infections. It may well be time for phages to take centre stage, not as a relic of medical history, but as a critical component of our future landscape.

Phages, with their precision targeting and natural abundance, might be what is needed in our fight against antibacterial resistance. In theory, phage therapy could well be a third arm of intervention after vaccines and antibiotics, especially as superbugs continue to rise. If we place a high value on protecting our microbiomes, then phage therapy might find a more significant place in mainstream medical practice too.

Vaccines

Vaccines prime the immune system to recognize and combat specific pathogens, such as bacteria or viruses. When introduced into the body, they stimulate the production of antibodies. Later, if the body is exposed to the actual pathogen, it's already equipped to defend against it.

Many bacterial vaccines are already available. For instance, vaccines for whooping cough and pneumococcus, a major cause of pneumonia and meningitis, are in use. For maximum benefit, vaccines should be widely administered since unvaccinated individuals represent a potential danger to the entire population.

We should intensify research to produce vaccines for the bacteria we currently can't combat. For instance, a universal vaccine against all strains of pneumococcus could diminish global antibiotic use, particularly in children under five who would otherwise be treated with antibiotics for pneumonia. Similarly, vaccines against bacteria like *Clostridium difficile*, certain carbapenem-resistant superbugs, and other superbugs in the Deadly Six could substantially decrease our dependency on antibiotics by thwarting infections before they occur.

Considering infections acquired in hospitals, some vaccines might be more beneficial for targeted populations rather than for the general public. However, people admitted to hospitals are at an elevated risk of contracting resistant infections, and they may benefit from additional immunity for the brief period that they are in hospital.

While vaccines have revolutionized public health, they aren't without challenges. Pathogens evolve, leading to 'vaccine escape' where they bypass the immunity provided by vaccines. However, such evolution in bacteria is less common than antibiotic resistance. Unlike antibiotics, vaccines don't exert direct selective pressure on the myriad microbes within our bodies.

A landmark study published in 2023 in the *BMJ Global Health* journal suggests vaccines might help to reduce the impact of superbugs. The primary benefit of vaccines is their ability to prevent infections before they even begin. Fewer people get sick and die. With fewer infections, there's also lesser need to use antibiotics. When we rely less on antibiotics, we reduce the chance of bugs evolving into superbugs.

This research, involving expert organizations like the WHO, finds that using specific vaccines could potentially prevent over half a million microbe-related deaths yearly. The study, which focused on fifteen vaccines targeting the most dangerous microbes, yielded impressive results. By using these vaccines strategically, we can not only save numerous lives but also drastically reduce the number of people suffering long-term health consequences from these infections. Two specific regions of the world, Africa and Southeast Asia, suffer the most from these vaccine-preventable infections.

The study suggests that these vaccines could significantly help these regions.

However, while vaccines are powerful tools, they can't be the only solution. If vaccines existed for all of the major superbugs, then we would have needed fewer antibiotics in the first place. In general, there are more vaccines that prevent viral infections than there are vaccines that prevent bacterial infections.

We can also fight superbugs by promoting vaccines that work against viral infections. Many illnesses caused by viruses often get treated with antibiotics due to symptom similarity or misdiagnosis. For example, rotavirus triggers a form of diarrhoea indistinguishable from some bacterial infections. Without swift diagnostic tools, antibiotics are frequently prescribed, and widespread use of the rotavirus vaccine could curb unwarranted antibiotic use.

Antimicrobial Peptides

All creatures, from tiny flies to humans, have immune systems to protect against infections. One of the frontline defenders of this system is a group of proteins called antimicrobial peptides. These proteins are everywhere in our bodies, particularly in areas where harmful germs could potentially enter, such as our skin and eyes. We're still trying to understand how these peptides work. For instance, we're not sure which germs they work best against, or if they work best on their own or in association with other peptides.

The history of our understanding of these natural products goes back to the late 1800s. Researchers found out that both human cells and certain moths produced low-weight proteins that played a crucial role in immunity. The most potent naturally occurring peptides we know of are from the horseshoe crab and pigs. Many of these antimicrobial peptides do more than just kill bacteria. They play a big role in the body's first line of defence. For instance, they can prevent bacteria from forming biofilms, which are shields that bacteria use to protect themselves. Some of these peptides, like ones derived from pigs, have strong effects against bacteria. And while some of these peptides work by breaking the bacteria's cell wall, others interfere with their inner processes.

But not all these natural peptides are very effective, and there are challenges, like for example, the body's natural salts can reduce their effectiveness. One of the challenges of developing these peptides as drugs is their cost and stability. They can also be easily broken down by enzymes in the body. However, scientists are finding ways around these challenges using computer modelling and biological engineering. This approach helps us understand the structure of the peptides and predict how they'll function.

Good Bacteria

Probiotics, often referred to as 'good bacteria', hold great promise in restoring our body's bacterial equilibrium. These beneficial microbes can offset the harmful effects of antibiotics by replenishing the beneficial bacteria that get depleted. Research indicates that probiotics can even limit the likelihood of certain post-antibiotic infections. However, not all probiotics are equally effective. While many can be beneficial, others offer no advantage, and in some rare situations, they may even be detrimental.

Imagine the human microbiome as a bustling city of microbes, where diversity ensures stability and health. A diverse microbiome is crucial for the optimal functioning of our immune system, with implications for weight control and susceptibility to various gastrointestinal conditions. As we age, natural shifts like reduced gastric acidity can perturb our microbiome. Consequently, older people are more prone to infections, especially after antibiotic usage.

So, faced with a disturbed microbiome, how do we repair it? A diverse microbiome can deter resistant pathogens by heightening the contest for essential resources. This quest brings the burgeoning science of microbiome-focused therapies to the forefront. While being especially beneficial for individuals frequently exposed to broad-spectrum antimicrobials, these therapies might render them less vulnerable to superbugs.

Two modern concepts in gut health are prebiotics and postbiotics. Prebiotics are specific food components that, while indigestible to us, provide nourishment for our beneficial gut bacteria. They are the special dishes that our gut bacteria thrive on. But not all prebiotics behave the same way. Some, especially when consumed in excessive amounts, might not be as beneficial as we think. A glaring example is certain purified soluble fibres, which when consumed excessively, could heighten the risk of diseases like liver cancer, especially if our gut health is already not at its best.

Dietary fibres are found predominantly in plant-based foods. Of special interest are plant polysaccharides, which are intricate networks of sugar molecules. Unlike sugars or starches, our bodies can't directly digest these complex fibres. But what's undigestible to us is a banquet for specialized gut bacteria, and these bacteria possess enzymes that break them down.

As these microbes feast upon and digest fibres, they release certain beneficial compounds (notably butyrate and propionate) called short-chain fatty acids, which are celebrated for a plethora of health benefits. Beyond their ability to curb inflammation, a root cause of numerous diseases, they play pivotal roles in strengthening our immune responses. They also influence cholesterol levels and even how full we feel after a meal, which can indirectly help in weight management.

Postbiotics are beneficial compounds that gut bacteria

produce as they metabolize their food sources. Short-chain fatty acids are one kind of postbiotic. The influence of postbiotics is not restricted to the gut as they act like messengers, conveying benefits throughout our body. For instance, butyrate travels and acts on specific receptors in our body, helping suppress inflammation and promote the growth and function of beneficial immune cells. Similarly, propionate is involved in sugar production in the liver and even plays a role in cholesterol management.

In addition, there is a close relationship between dietary fibres and gut bacteria. Specific types of fibres favour the growth of particular bacteria. For example, a fibre known as resistant starch acts as a magnet for a bacteria called *Eubacterium rectale*. In contrast, another variety seems to be the preferred meal for *Parabacteroides distasonis*. This predictability in how fibres influence bacterial communities opens the possibility of customizing our diets based on unique gut microbiomes to unlock optimal health benefits.

However, as far as fibre is concerned, more isn't always better. You might assume that gobbling down heaps of fibre will directly translate to better gut health, but that's a simplistic notion. If our resident bacteria have already reached their full capacity in processing fibre, adding more won't necessarily boost short-chain fatty acid production.

There's another approach to restoring the gut microbiome to its former state which involves introducing good bacteria from others. Our minds are primed to recoil at the thought of anything associated with faeces, which is universally seen as dirty and harmful. However, the medical world is finding benefits in the use of faecal material to treat certain intractable bacterial infections that cannot be treated with antibiotics. The technique, known as faecal microbiota transplantation (FMT), harnesses the power of a healthy person's stool to restore balance to the bacteria in a sick person's gut.

As we discussed in Chapter 8, various factors, especially the overuse of antibiotics, can disrupt this delicate balance of the gut microbiome. Such disruptions can make our bodies vulnerable to opportunistic pathogens. An example is *Clostridioides difficile*. It can overrun the gut, especially after antibiotic treatment, leading to severe diarrhoea and even life-threatening inflammation of the colon. This is where FMT is useful. By introducing a mixture of beneficial bacteria from a healthy person's stool into the gut of a patient with a disrupted microbiome, the balance can potentially be restored. The introduced bacteria can reset the ecosystem by outcompeting harmful ones.

In the case of *Clostridioides difficile* infections, the success rate of this procedure has been remarkable, with many patients showing significant improvement. Beyond *Clostridioides difficile*, there's growing interest in exploring FMT for other conditions like inflammatory bowel diseases, obesity, and even neurological disorders. The idea is that by modulating the gut's microbial community, it might be possible to influence other aspects of health.

However, FMT isn't entirely free from complications. One of the prime concerns is of safety. Transferring biological material between humans poses many risks. A thorough screening of the donor's stool is of paramount importance to ensure no harmful pathogens or substances are introduced into the recipient. But despite rigorous checks, there have been cases where individuals contracted infections post-transplantation due to unscreened or inadequately screened samples.

Beyond immediate safety issues, there's uncharted territory regarding the long-term implications of the procedure. While patients might experience quick relief from specific conditions, the broader, lasting impacts on their health are yet to be fully understood. For instance, a compelling area of study is the gut–brain axis, which highlights the potential influence of gut microbes on our mental well-being. As our understanding deepens, questions arise: by altering the gut's microbial community, are we inadvertently affecting neurological health? What might the long-term mental and emotional ramifications be?

Adding to the complexity is the inherent variability in our microbiomes. Just as no two individuals share the exact DNA, our microbial compositions are also distinct. This uniqueness poses challenges in ensuring that the donor's microbial profile aligns well with the recipient's needs. A transplant that proves beneficial for one patient might not necessarily provide the same results in another, making the pursuit of an ideal microbial match necessary but challenging.

Ethical considerations also complicate the landscape. While the medical benefits of FMT are apparent, the idea of transferring faecal matter, even when rigorously processed, can be a sensitive topic for many. Ensuring patients are adequately informed and understand the procedure's intricacies is vital. The balance between potential benefits and ethical concerns must be navigated delicately, emphasizing transparent communication and informed consent.

A longer-term goal in the emerging area of microbiome engineering would be to harness the potential of our own microbiomes to fight infections. Researchers are exploring the compounds produced by our gut bacteria, and these substances might hold the key to new treatments for certain infections.

Imagine bacteria custom-engineered to produce therapeutic compounds directly in our gut, acting as tiny factories that produce drugs inside us. Scientists are also working on cultivating specific beneficial bacterial strains. These lab-grown communities could then be introduced to patients, offering a more standardized and controlled approach than direct stool transplants. Although these approaches might sound like science fiction today, they could be in the realm of standard medical practice in a decade.

We must think beyond antibiotics to fight superbugs.

Diversifying our strategies is key to defeating antibiotic resistance. Exploring phages, vaccines, antimicrobial peptides and bolstering 'good bacteria' are some of the exciting ways we can tip the balance in our favour in the coming years.

15

The Hidden Pandemic

The story of antibiotics is a cautionary tale of a huge scientific triumph followed by great complacency. Today, antibiotic resistance is a silent, hidden pandemic, with profound consequences for global health. The main causes behind the rise of superbugs are complex and multifaceted. Between 2000 and 2015, there was a startling 65 per cent increase in antibiotic usage, particularly in low- and middle-income countries. This surge has inadvertently given bacteria ample opportunities to develop resistance and become superbugs, which spread seamlessly through humans, animals, and even the environment. And poor access to water, sanitation, and hygiene only exacerbates this situation.

A stark illustration of this menace can be seen among the most vulnerable section of any population – our infants. Infectious diseases remain a leading cause of death for children under five. Globally, over 210,000 infant deaths are annually attributed to drug-resistant septic infections. And when you dig deeper, studies highlight that just one superbug, the antibiotic-resistant *Klebsiella pneumoniae*, contributes to mortality rates of 10–12 per cent among newborns with sepsis.

In India, more than half the strains of *Klebsiella pneumoniae* are already resistant to last-line antibiotics, making the situation particularly alarming – infants who pick up this this superbug often have no chance.

Moreover, the misuse of antibiotics isn't limited to hospitals. In the community, unwarranted prescriptions abound. A 2023 study of fifty-nine low- and medium-income countries published in the *eClinicalMedicine* journal found that a staggering three of four children reporting fever and cough were prescribed antibiotics. However, calling antibiotic resistance only a medical issue undersells its magnitude. It's an overarching public health crisis bridging human, agricultural, and environmental realms.

So, where might solutions lie? One promising avenue is the advent of rapid diagnostic tests. These revolutionary tools have the potential to not only pinpoint the microbial culprit behind infections, but also to indicate its resistance profile within hours. Such precision would empower clinicians to streamline treatments, reducing the reliance on broad-spectrum antibiotics.

But other challenges continue to persist. The identification of disease-causing microbes can still take days, making rapid diagnostic tools a luxury in many scenarios, especially in resource-poor settings. The result is that many healthcare providers resort to treatments based on symptoms rather than confirmed diagnosis. Even when physicians are aware of the limitations of antibiotics, the pressures of patient expectations or perceived caution can skew their judgement.

Further, the problem is compounded by the preventative use of antibiotics, often done to mask the lack of sanitation or to ward off potential secondary infections. These prescriptions for antibiotics are inappropriate for treating conditions like viral respiratory tract infections, which account for a significant percentage of antibiotic misuse.

Historically, prescribing antibiotics for a week or longer was common, often due to the need to be safe. Today, despite guidelines recommending shorter treatment periods, many infections like community acquired pneumonia are still treated for ten days or longer, exposing patients to unnecessary risks.

Combating superbugs requires understanding how resistance develops through interactions among bacteria, their hosts, the environment, and human interventions. What we need to talk about more, however, is the environmental dimension of antimicrobial resistance. Antibiotics don't magically disappear after they've served their purpose in medicine or agriculture. They persist in our waterways and soil, creating environments where only the fittest, most resistant, superbugs thrive. The consequences of our choices today will be suffered by future generations – the very medicines designed to save lives today could be shaping an ecosystem hostile to life in the long term.

The intricate relationship between bacteria and their environments significantly impacts our health and well-being. Far from being isolated entities, bacteria continually swap genes, a process that has the potential to turn harmless strains into undefeatable superbugs. The superbug crisis is further heightened by our planet's changing climate. As global temperatures rise, so does the speed at which bacteria replicate, perpetuating a cycle where the demand for effective antibiotics surges while their efficacy falls.

Addressing this multidimensional issue demands a holistic approach that incorporates human, animal, and environmental health. We must embrace the idea that our well-being is intrinsically tied to the health of animals and our shared environment.

Every facet of life on Earth, from our health to our food sources and even our ecosystems, is currently being imperilled. Bacteria are adapting to the world as we change it, and we are heading closer to a post-antibiotic era where even the simplest infections are deadly. Confronting this adaptive challenge mandates that we, too, evolve in our response, to protect antibiotics as a shared, societal resource. We must understand that the problem of superbugs isn't just an issue of health but a deeper socio-economic one. In many countries, packed cities grow even further, and a combination of poor sanitation, low-quality water, and poor hygiene increases the spread of superbugs.

A growing area of concern is the rise in antibiotic resistance within livestock such as chickens, cows, and pigs. Consuming these animals transfers the resistant bacteria into our systems. Yet, animals aren't solely the cause of such transmissions. Humans, often guilty of antibiotic misuse, can inadvertently transfer these resistant strains back to the animal kingdom. This mutual exchange, which is particularly rampant in environments with subpar hygiene and lax safety measures, only exacerbates the situation.

Poor water and waste management systems, especially in developing nations, worsen the situation. The proximity of waste dumps to residential and farming areas can result in antibiotic-resistant bacterial contamination of water sources and food. Even seemingly inconspicuous entities, like flies, can serve as carriers and spread these bacteria.

Superbugs know no boundaries. Given the ubiquity of international travel and commerce, antibiotic resistance has transcended continents, making it a global concern. Consider the vibrant cattle trade between India and Bangladesh, valued at over US$600 million annually. Much of this trade bypasses official channels, eschewing crucial safety checks. This pattern mirrors the ones in countries like Nigeria, where a sizeable chunk of the poultry trade follows an informal trajectory. Coupled with scant access to veterinarians in some regions, antibiotic misuse runs rampant.

The interplay between poverty, infectious diseases, and antibiotic resistance forms a self-perpetuating cycle. Those in poverty are disproportionately affected by infectious diseases. The contributing factors are many – overcrowded living conditions, insufficient nutrition, lack of access to clean water, and inadequate healthcare. These conditions not only facilitate the spread of infections but also create environments in which diseases flourish.

As infectious diseases take hold, the economic burden they impose can be crushing. The costs associated with medical treatment, coupled with the loss of income during illness, perpetuate poverty. Complicating this issue is the pervasive spread of antibiotic resistance, a dire consequence that emerges from the depths of poverty. In areas where healthcare systems are strained and health education is lacking, antibiotics are often misused, whether through incomplete courses of treatment or unregulated distribution.

The result is a harrowing cycle where the consequences of illness serve to reinforce the impoverished conditions that initially made individuals vulnerable. Breaking this cycle requires more than just medical intervention; it requires improving sanitation and access to healthcare and encouraging responsible antibiotic use along with socio-economic support.

Addressing this challenge requires customized solutions that resonate with the unique challenges of communities. At a basic level, we should prioritize solutions like improving sanitation and hygiene. The COVID-19 pandemic made people aware of the importance of these solutions in disease prevention, and we must capitalize on this momentum.

Through this book, we've tried to uncover the root causes behind the rise of superbugs and explored a series of possible solutions to the challenges they pose. Central to our discussion is the urgent need to restrict the use of vital antibiotics, particularly those that are indispensable to healthcare. Advocating for their prohibition in agricultural practices, and curbing their release into the environment are steps we must consider. In parallel, a shift in our medical application of antibiotics is necessary. Emphasizing both careful prescription and innovative treatments, we can ensure antibiotics remain effective for longer.

A core initiative in this process is antibiotic stewardship. This principle champions a thoughtful approach to antibiotic prescription, echoing the caution we exercise with our valuable resources. By ensuring that antibiotics are prescribed only when crucially required and then only in the correct fashion, we can mitigate potential side effects. The vigilant monitoring of certain antibiotics, known to induce specific infections, is also essential. Further, some healthcare centres have adopted a rotation method for antibiotics in the hope of counteracting bacterial resistance.

Using a targeted treatment strategy is another solution that's gaining traction. Drawing inspiration from the precision of missiles, the aim is to deliver medications tailored to the microbe without causing unnecessary collateral damage. This ensures that antibiotics target only specific parts of the body.

The goal is also to tailor treatments to neutralize specific detrimental bacteria while sparing the harmless ones. Current scientific explorations are also venturing into the realm of utilizing natural agents like phages, which demonstrate pinpointed destructive capabilities against certain bacteria. However, for such treatments to be effective, clinicians must identify the offending bacteria, a determination that may be difficult to achieve in practice at scale.

What is abundantly clear is that inaction is not an option. We must acknowledge that while the world grappled with the COVID-19 pandemic, a quieter, but no less deadly, pandemic had also been brewing.

Despite all of these challenges, I am hopeful. Humans are capable of rising up to challenges once we acknowledge their existence. We may not have the same antibiotics and antibacterial drugs we do today, but twenty years from now, I believe we will have new tools to wage our continuing war against superbugs.

Additional Resources

Reading

McKenna, Maryn. 2018. *Plucked! The Truth About Chicken.* New York: Little, Brown.

Hall, William, Anthony McDonnell and Jim O'Neill. 2018. *Superbugs: An Arms Race against Bacteria.* Boston: Harvard University Press.

Strathdee, Steffanie and Thomas Patterson. 2020. *The Perfect Predator: A Scientist's Race to Save Her Husband from a Deadly Superbug.* New York: Hachette Books.

Viewing

FRONTLINE. 'When Antibiotics Don't Work (Full Documentary) | Frontline.' YouTube, 22 December 2021. https://www.youtube.com/watch?v=EkyAuG9RSSU.

Wright, Gerry. 'How Can We Solve the Antibiotic Resistance Crisis? – Ted-Ed.' YouTube, 16 March 2020. https://www.youtube.com/watch?v=ZvhFeGEDFC8.

Al Jazeera English. 'The Rise of India's Superbugs | 101 East.'

YouTube, 17 August 2016. https://www.youtube.com/watch?v=ofbtepraOX4.
Wech, Michael, dir. *Silent Pandemic*. Broadview Pictures, in co-production with ZDF and in cooperation with ARTE. Cologne, Germany, 2022. https://www.amr-film.com/synopsis/.

Listening

'The Evidence: Drug-resistant Superbugs,' *The Discovery* (podcast), 26 February 2022. https://www.bbc.co.uk/programmes/p0br7g3h.
'The Inquiry: How Did We Mess up Antibiotics?,' *The Inquiry* (podcast), 6 April 2019, https://www.bbc.co.uk/programmes/p04bnkjr.
Superbugs & You (podcast series): https://www.cidrap.umn.edu/antimicrobial-stewardship/superbugs-you.
'Discovering New Antibiotics,' *Editors in Conversation* (podcast), 5 October 2020, https://asm.org/Podcasts/Editors-in-Conversation/Episodes/Discovering-new-antibiotics-EIC-9.

Notes

This book was developed through extensive research involving over five hundred sources including books, scientific articles, reviews, news reports, and multimedia materials. Given the vast array of resources, it is impractical to list each one. This is a curated selection of the most relevant references.

Preface

1 **In India alone**... Nogrady, B. 'The Fight against Antimicrobial Resistance'. *Nature*, no. 624 (7991): 30–32, 2023. DOI: 10.1038/d41586-023-03912-8.
2 **The last new major class of antibiotics** ... Hutchings, M., A. Truman, and B. Wilkinson. 'Antibiotics: Past, Present and Future.' *Current Opinion in Microbiology*, 51: 72–80, 2019. Preprint at https://doi.org/10.1016/j.mib.2019.10.008.
3 **No truly innovative antibiotics**... The Pew Charitable Trusts. 'Researcher Explains Challenges in Finding Novel Antibiotics.' The Pew Charitable Trusts, 18 February 2021. https://www.pewtrusts.org/en/research-and-analysis/articles/2021/02/18/researcher-explains-challenges-in-finding-novel-antibiotics.

4. **Table modified from data** ... Coque, T. M. et al. 'Strengthening Environmental Action in the One Health Response to Antimicrobial Resistance'. United Nations Environment Programme, 2023. https://www.unep.org/resources/superbugs/environmental-action.

5. **More recently around 60–80 per cent of patients** ... Malik, S.S. and S. Mundra. 'Increasing Consumption of Antibiotics during the COVID-19 Pandemic: Implications for Patient Health and Emerging Anti-Microbial Resistance.' *Antibiotics*, no. 12(1): 45, 2023. DOI: 10.3390/antibiotics12010045.

6. **Even if physicians suspected** ... Alshaikh, F.S., et al. 'Prevalence of Bacterial Coinfection and Patterns of Antibiotics Prescribing in Patients with COVID-19: A Systematic Review and Meta-Analysis.' *PLoS One* 17, no. 8: e0272375, 2022. DOI: 10.1371/journal.pone.0272375.

1. A Daily Tragedy

1. **'As a mother, you feel so helpless** ... Melhem, Yaara Bou. 'What Is Killing India's Babies?' Al Jazeera, 15 August 2016. https://www.aljazeera.com/features/2016/8/15/what-is-killing-indias-babies.

2. **Anjali's daughter is one of the approximately** ... Williams, P. C.M. et al. 'Antibiotics Needed to Treat Multidrug-Resistant Infections in Neonates.' *Bull World Health Organ*, no. 100: 797–807, 2022. DOI: 10.2471/BLT.22.288623.

3. **Consider this** ... O'Neill, Aaron. 'India: Life Expectancy 1800–2020.' Statista, 21 June 2022. https://www.statista.com/statistics/1041383/life-expectancy-india-all-time/.

4 **Natural selection of Antibiotic-Resistant Bacteria...** ReAct Group. 'Mutations and Selection – Antibiotic Resistance.' ReAct, 26 January 2023. https://www.reactgroup.org/toolbox/understand/antibiotic-resistance/mutation-and-selection/.

5 **'Evolution is cleverer...** Dunitz, Jack D. and Gerald F. Joyce. National Academy of Sciences, 2013. 'Leslie E. Orgel: Biographical Memoirs.' https://www.nasonline.org/publications/biographical-memoirs/memoir-pdfs/orgel-leslie.pdf.

6 **In August of that year...** Kumarasamy, K.K. et al. 'Emergence of a New Antibiotic Resistance Mechanism in India, Pakistan, and the UK: A Molecular, Biological, and Epidemiological Study.' *The Lancet Infectious Diseases*, 9, no. 10: 597–602, 2010.

7 **The second spark...** O'Neill, J.T. 'Tackling Drug-Resistance Infections Globally: Final Report and Recommendations,' 2016. The Review on Antimicrobial Resistance. Available at: https://amr-review.org/.

8 **The World Health Organization (WHO) estimates that...** World Health Organization. '14.9 Million Excess Deaths Associated with the COVID-19 Pandemic in 2020 and 2021.' https://www.who.int/news/item/05-05-2022-14.9-million-excess-deaths-were-associated-with-the-covid-19-pandemic-in-2020-and-2021.

9 **If the O'Neill report which outlined...** Murray, C.J. et al. 'Global Burden of Bacterial Antimicrobial Resistance in 2019: A Systematic Analysis.' *The Lancet*, 399, no. 10325: 629–55, 2022. DOI: https://doi.org/10.1016/S0140-6736(21)02724-0.

Notes

2. Superbug Signatures

1   **How Bacteria Share Their Superpowers . . .** Centers for Disease Control and Prevention. 'Antibiotic/Antimicrobial Resistance: Fact Sheets'. Available at: https://www.cdc.gov/drugresistance/resources/fact-sheets.html.
2   **In fact, Alexander Fleming . . .** Fleming, Alexander. 'The Nobel Prize in Physiology or Medicine 1945.' NobelPrize.org. https://www.nobelprize.org/prizes/medicine/1945/fleming/lecture/.

3. Blindness in a Bottle

1   **In early 2023, a chilling story . . .** ASM.org. 'A Dangerous Eye Infection from Tainted Eye Drops, Months Before the CDC's Warning'. https://asm.org/Press-Releases/2023/May/A-dangerous-eye-infection-from-tainted-eye-drops,.
2   **All fingers pointed to a common source . . .** CBC News. 'How U.S. Officials Solved the Mystery of Eyedrops Infecting Dozens with Drug-Resistant Bacteria'. https://www.cbc.ca/news/health/eyedrops-us-bacteria-1.6762792.
3   **Around 13 per cent of *Pseudomonas* . . .** Horcajada, J.P. et al. 'Epidemiology and Treatment of Multidrug-Resistant and Extensively Drug-Resistant *Pseudomonas aeruginosa* Infections.' *Clinical Microbiology Reviews*, 34, no. 4, 2019. DOI: 10.1128/CMR.00031-19.
4   **What set this outbreak apart . . .** Bartels, Meghan. 'Eye Drops Recalled after Deaths and Blindness – Here's What to Know.' *Scientific American*, 24 March 2023. https://www.scientificamerican.com/article/eye-drops-recalled-after-deaths-and-blindness-heres-what-to-know/.

5   **Unfortunately, what the CDC had spotted . . .** Centers for Disease Control and Prevention, 18 May 2023. https://www.cdc.gov/hai/outbreaks/crpa-artificial-tears.html#anchor_1674746879046.

6   **What this means was the strain . . .** Morelli, M.K. et al. 'Investigating and Treating a Corneal Ulcer Due to Extensively Drug-Resistant *Pseudomonas aeruginosa*.' *Antimicrobial Agents and Chemotherapy*, 67, no. 7, 2023. https://journals.asm.org/doi/full/10.1128/aac.00277-23.

7   **The two key enzymes that the deadly superbug made . . .** Centers for Disease Control and Prevention, 18 May 2023. https://www.cdc.gov/hai/outbreaks/crpa-artificial-tears.html#anchor_1674746879046.

8   **On the other hand, the GES . . .** Poirel, L. et al. 'Biochemical Sequence Analyses of GES-1 – A Novel Class A Extended-spectrum β-lactamase, and the Class 1 integron In52 from *Klebsiella pneumoniae*.' *Antimicrobial Agents and Chemotherapy*, 44, no. 3: 622–32, 2000.

9   **At this point, all signs . . .** Holpuch, Amanda. 'Eye Drops Are Recalled after Being Linked to Vision Loss and 1 Death.' *New York Times*, 2 February 2023. https://www.nytimes.com/2023/02/02/business/eye-drops-ezricare-infections-cdc.html.

10 **And tragically, the outbreak resulted . . .** 'Outbreak of Extensively Drug-Resistant *Pseudomonas aeruginosa* Associated with Artificial Tears.' Centers for Disease Control and Prevention, 18 May 2023. https://www.cdc.gov/hai/outbreaks/crpa-artificial-tears.html#anchor_1674746879046.

11 **Consider the ordeal of . . .** Jewett, Christina and Andrew Jacobs. 'Drug-Resistant Bacteria Tied to Eyedrops Can Spread Person

to Person.' *New York Times*, 3 April 2023. https://www.nytimes.com/2023/04/03/health/superbug-eyedrops-blindness.html.

12 **Bloomberg reported that** . . . Bloomberg. 'No Testing, No Inspections: Contaminated Eyedrops Blinded and Killed Americans.' https://www.bloomberg.com/news/features/2023-07-17/eyedrop-recall-2023-and-infections-were-result-of-lack-of-fda-regulation?embedded-checkout=true.

13 **In a story published in** . . . Jewett, Christina and Andrew Jacobs. 'Drug-Resistant Bacteria Tied to Eyedrops Can Spread Person to Person.' *New York Times*, 3 April 2023. https://www.nytimes.com/2023/04/03/health/superbug-eyedrops-blindness.html.

14 **On 27 October** . . . US Food and Drug Administration. 'FDA Warns Consumers Not to Purchase Or Use Certain Eye Drops from Several Major Brands Due to Risk of Eye Infection.' https://www.fda.gov/drugs/drug-safety-and-availability/fda-warns-consumers-not-purchase-or-use-certain-eye-drops-several-major-brands-due-risk-eye.

15 **All bacteria have genes that produce proteins** . . . Smith, W.P.J. et al. 'Bacterial Defences: Mechanisms, Evolution and Antimicrobial Resistance.' *Nature Reviews Microbiology*, 21: 519–34, 2023.

16 **Some bacteria produce enzymes that** . . . Darby, E.M. et al. 'Molecular Mechanisms of Antibiotic Resistance Revisited.' *Nature Reviews Microbiology*, 21: 280–95, 2023.

4. The New Delhi Story

1 **The controversy was sparked by** . . . Kumarasamy, K.K. et al. 'Emergence of a New Antibiotic Resistance Mechanism

Notes

in India, Pakistan, and the UK: A Molecular, Biological, and Epidemiological Study.' *The Lancet Infectious Diseases*, 9, no. 10: 597–602, 2010.

2 **According to contemporaneous media reports** ... Iyenger, P. Chennai Corner. *Outlook*, 18 August 2010. https://www.outlookindia.com/amp/story/national/chennai-corner-news-266783.

3 **The editor-in-chief of the parent journal** ... Sinha, Kounteya. 'Lancet Says Sorry for "Delhi Bug".' *Times of India*, 12 January 2011. https://timesofindia.indiatimes.com/india/lancet-says-sorry-for-delhi-bug/articleshow/7261135.cms.

4 **Later, one of the lead authors claimed** ... McKenna, M. *Plucked! The Truth about Chicken*. Little, Brown, 2017.

5 **A decade later, while giving** ... Walsh, Timothy. 'Mechanisms of Antibiotic Resistance: What Makes a Superbug? | Professor Timothy Walsh.' YouTube, 18 June 2019. https://www.youtube.com/watch?v=HZriDiN4T_o.

6 **Much of the angst in India** ... Mohapatra, P.R. 'Metallo-β-lactamase 1 – Why Blame New Delhi & India?' *Indian Journal of Medical Research*, 137, no. 1: 213–15, 2013.

7 **In 2021, an editorial in** ... Editorial. 'The Lancet Infectious Diseases. An Eventful 20 Years.' *The Lancet Infectious Diseases*, 21, no. 8: 1051, 2021.

8 **In fact, the discovery of the resistance gene** ... Yong, D. et al. 'Characterization of a New Metallo-β-lactamase gene, bla(NDM-1), in *Klebsiella pneumoniae* ST14 from India.' *Antimicrobial Agents and Chemotherapy*, 53, no. 12: 5046–54, 2009.

9 **It is an enzyme encoded by** ... Conventionally, bacterial resistance genes are written in italics and lowercase letters to differentiate them from the proteins they encode.

Notes

10 **But carbapenemases have an extensive 'toolkit'** ... Arias, C.A. and B.E. Murray. 'Antibiotic-Resistant Bugs in the 21st Century – A Clinical Super-Challenge.' *The New England Journal of Medicine*, 360: 439–43, 2009.

11 **Later in 2009, a team of researchers** ... Deshpande, P. et al. 'New Delhi Metallo-Beta Lactamase (Ndm-1) in Enterobacteriaceae: Treatment Options with Carbapenems Compromised.' *Journal of the Association of Physicians of India*, 58: 147–49, 2010.

12 **According to multiple media outlets** ... Agence France-Presse. '"New Delhi" Superbug Stigmatized a Single Country and City': Medical ...' *National Post*, 13 January 2011. https://nationalpost.com/health/new-delhi-superbug-stigmatized-a-single-country-and-city-medical-journal-editor/.

13 **The WHO advises against associating viruses** ... Kupferschmidt, K. 'Discovered a Disease? WHO Has New Rules for Avoiding Offensive Names.' *Science*, 2015. https://www.science.org/content/article/discovered-disease-who-has-new-rules-avoiding-offensive-names.

14 **It is also important to note the stance** ... Government of India. 'Reported NDM-1 not a Significant Problem: Min of H&FW.' 2011. Available at: https://www.pib.gov.in/newsite/PrintRelease.aspx?relid=71532.

15 **A perspective published in the leading medical journal** ... Moellering, R.C. 'NDM-1 – A Cause for Worldwide Concern.' *The New England Journal of Medicine*, 363: 2377–79, 2010.

16 **In 2011, the next chapter of the saga** ... Walsh, T.R. et al. 'Dissemination of NDM-1 Positive Bacteria in New Delhi.' *The Lancet Infectious Diseases*, 11, no. 5: 355–62, 2011.

17 **By 2017, things took another twist** ... Khan, A.U. et al. 'Structure, Genetics, and Spread of New Delhi Metallo-β-

lactamase (NDM).' *BMC Microbiology*, 17: 1–12, 2017. Preprint at https://doi.org/10.1186/s12866-017-1012-8.

18 **A report in the scientific journal *PLoS Medicine* ...** Walsh, T.R. et al. 'Antimicrobial Resistance: Addressing a Global Threat to Humanity.' *PLoS Medicine*, 20, no. 7: e1004264, 2023. Preprint at https://doi.org/10.1371/journal.pmed.1004264.

5. The Last Line Falls

1 **More than seven decades after the discovery of colistin ...** Sabnis, A. et al. 'Colistin Kills Bacteria by Targeting Lipopolysaccharide in the Cytoplasmic Membrane.' *eLife* 10: e65836, 2021.

2 ***Pseudomonas* infections are amongst the most common ...** Centers for Disease Control and Prevention. *Pseudomonas aeruginosa Infection*. Available at: https://www.cdc.gov/hai/organisms/pseudomonas.html.

3 **A new resistance gene was identified in a pig ...** Liu, Y.Y. et al. 'Emergence of Plasmid-Mediated Colistin Resistance Mechanism MCR-1 in China.' *The Lancet Infectious Diseases*, 16, no. 2: 161–68, 2016.

4 **What makes MCR-1 particularly alarming ...** Centers for Disease Control and Prevention. *Newly Reported Gene, mcr-1, Threatens Last-Resort Antibiotics*. Available at: https://www.cdc.gov/drugresistance/solutions-initiative/stories/gene-reported-mcr.html.

5 **Between 2011 and 2014 ...** Liu, Y.Y. et al. Emergence of plasmid-mediated colistin resistance mechanism MCR-1 in China. *The Lancet Infectious Diseases*, 16: 161–68, 2016.

6 **By 2017, research by various scientists had delved deeper ...** Quan, J. et al. 'Prevalence of MCR-1 in *Escherichia coli* and

Klebsiella pneumoniae in China.' *The Lancet Infectious Diseases*, 17, no. 4: 400–10, 2017.

7 **A 2018 study revealed a global picture** . . . Wang, R. et al. 'The Global Distribution and Spread of the Mobilized Colistin Resistance Gene MCR-1.' *Nature Communications*, 9: 1–9, 2018.

8 **In 2022, a comprehensive analysis** . . . Binsker, U., A.K. Asbohrer and J.A. Hammerl. 'Global Colistin Use and Resistant Enterobacterales.' *FEMS Microbiology Reviews*, 46: 1–37, 2022.

9 **A detailed analysis in the journal** *Pathogens* . . . Bastidas-Caldes, C. et al. 'Worldwide Prevalence of MCR-mediated Colistin-Resistance *Escherichia coli*.' *Pathogens*, 11, no. 6, 2022. DOI: 10.3390/pathogens11060659.

10 **An investigative report brought to light** . . . The Bureau of Investigative Journalism. 'A Game of Chicken: How Indian Poultry Farming is Creating Global Superbugs.' https://www.thebureauinvestigates.com/stories/2018-01-30/a-game-of-chicken-how-indian-poultry-farming-is-creating-global-superbugs.

11 **India was spurred into action** . . . The Bureau of Investigative Journalism. 'India bans use of "last hope" antibiotic on farms.' https://www.thebureauinvestigates.com/stories/2019-07-22/india-bans-use-of-last-hope-antibiotic-colistin-on-farms.

6. The Eye of the Storm

1 **The researchers combined antibiotic consumption** . . . Klein, E.Y., et al. 'Tracking Global Trends in the Effectiveness of Antibiotic Therapy Using the Drug Resistance Index.' *BMJ Global Health* 4, no. 2: e001315, 2019.

2 **A news story summarized the findings** ... Laha, Moumita. 'India Tops the List of Countries with Highest Antibiotic Resistance, Finds Study.' Research Matters, 10 September 2019. https://researchmatters.in/news/india-tops-list-countries-highest-antibiotic-resistance-finds-study.

3 **We can argue the merits of the approach** ... Vandenbroucke-Grauls, C.M. J.E. et al. 'The Proposed Drug Resistance Index (DRI) Is Not a Good Measure of Antibiotic Effectiveness in Relation to Drug Resistance.' *BMJ Global Health*, 4, no. 4: e001838, 2019.

4 **Earlier, in 2017, the same organization** ... Gandra, S., J. Joshi, A. Trett and A. Sankhil-Lamkang. *Scoping Report on Antimicrobial Resistance in India*. Center for Disease Dynamics, Economics & Policy, 1–130, 2017.

5 **India isn't only the world's most populous nation** ... Fazaludeen Koya, S. et al. 'Antibiotic Consumption in India: Geographical Variations and Temporal Changes between 2011 and 2019.' *JAC-Antimicrobal Resistance*, 4, no. 5, 2022. DOI: 10.1093/jacamr/dlac112.

6 **In fact, India single-handedly** ... McGettigan, P., Peter Roderick, Abhay Kadam and Allyson Pollock. 'Threats to Global Antimicrobial Resistance Control: Centrally Approved and Unapproved Antibiotic Formulations Sold in India.' *British Journal of Clinical Pharmacology*, 85, no. 1: 59–70.

7 **One study estimated that just under half** ... Kotwani, A. and K. Holloway. 'Trends in Antibiotic Use Among Outpatients in New Delhi, India.' *BMC Infectious Diseases*, 11: 1–9, 2011.

8 **A significant portion of the antibiotics** ... Koya, S.F. et al. 'Consumption of Systemic Antibiotics in India in 2019.' *The Lancet Regional Health Southeast Asia*, 4: 100025, 2022.

9   **Within the established confines of hospitals** . . . Nogrady, B. 'The Fight against Antimicrobial Resistance.' *Nature*, no. 624 (7991): 30–32, 2023. DOI: 10.1038/d41586-023-03912-8.
10 **They can treat bacterial co-infections** . . . Morens, D.M., J.K. Taubenberger and A.S. Fauci. 'Predominant Role of Bacterial Pneumonia as a Cause of Death in Pandemic Influenza: Implications for Pandemic Influenza Preparedness.' *The Journal of Infectious Diseases*, 198, no. 7: 962–70, 2008.
11 **There's research showing that around** . . . Cong, W. et al. 'Antimicrobial Use in COVID-19 Patients in the First Phase of the SARS-CoV-2 Pandemic: A Scoping Review.' *Antibiotics* (Basel), 10, no. 6: 745, 2021.
12 **The Indian Council of Medical Research (ICMR), through** . . . Indian Council of Medical Research. *AMRSN Annual Report 2022*. https://main.icmr.nic.in/sites/default/files/guidelines/AMRSN_Annual_Report_2022.pdf.
13 **Compared with other similar-sized economies** . . . Petrie, D., and K.K. Tang. 'Relative Health Performance in Brics over the Past 20 Years: The Winners and Losers.' *Bulletin of the World Health Organization*, 92, no. 6: 396–404, 2014.

7. The World Outside

1   **A landmark study traced this superbug's lineage** . . . Larsen, J. et al. 'Emergence of Methicillin Resistance Predates the Clinical Use of Antibiotics.' *Nature*, 602: 135–41, 2022.
2   **As Ewan Harrison, a senior author of the study** . . . University of Oxford. 'Superbug MRSA Arose in Hedgehogs Long Before Clinical Use of Antibiotics'. 5 January 2022. https://www.ox.ac.uk/news/2022-01-05-superbug-mrsa-arose-hedgehogs-long-clinical-use-antibiotics.

3   **We should remember that some form of resistance . . .** Wright, G.D. 'The Antibiotic Resistome: The Nexus of Chemical and Genetic Diversity.' *Nature Reviews Microbiology*, 5: 175–86, 2007. Preprint at https://doi.org/10.1038/nrmicro1614.

4   **In the wild, the usage of antibiotics greatly . . .** Spagnolo, F., M. Trujillo and J.J. Dennehy. 'Why Do Antibiotics Exist?' *mBio*, 12, no. 6, 2021. DOI: 10.1128/mBio.01966-21.

5   **Casting the net wider could help us to . . .** Clardy, J., M.A. Fischbach and C.R. Currie. 'The Natural History of Antibiotics.' *Current Biology*, 19, no. 11: 437–41, 2009. Preprint at https://doi.org/10.1016/j.cub.2009.04.001.

6   **Extracting DNA directly from environmental samples . . .** Hover, B.M. et al. 'Culture-Independent Discovery of the Malacidins as Calcium-Dependent Antibiotics with Activity against Multidrug-Resistant Gram-Positive Pathogens.' *Nature Microbiology*, 3: 415–22, 2018.

8. The World Within Us

1   **You see, antibiotics don't discriminate . . .** de Nies, L., C.M. Kobras and M. Stracy. 'Antibiotic-induced Collateral Damage to the Microbiota and Associated Infections.' *Nature Reviews Microbiology*, 21: 789–804, 2023. Preprint at https://doi.org/10.1038/s41579-023-00936-9.

2   **A common side effect of antibiotics is diarrhoea, occurring, by some estimates . . .** Mekonnen, S.A., D. Merenstein, C.M. Fraser and M.L. Marco. 'Molecular Mechanisms of Probiotic Prevention of Antibiotic-Associated Diarrhea.' *Current Opinion in Biotechnology*, 61: 226–34, 2020.

3   Among those who later developed ... Marshall, C. and E. McBryde. 'The Role of *Staphylococcus aureus* Carriage in the Pathogenesis of Bloodstream Infection.' *BMC Research Notes*, 7: 1–6, 2014.

9. How We Stumbled on Antibiotics (and Resistance)

1   Researchers have found traces of tetracycline ... Aminov, R.I. 'A Brief History of the Antibiotic Era: Lessons Learned and Challenges for the Future.' *Frontiers in Microbiology*, 2010. DOI: 10.3389/fmicb.2010.00134.
2   Referring to them as 'little animals' ... Snyder, Laura J. 'A Kingdom of Little Animals.' *The American Scholar*, 1 June 2013. https://theamericanscholar.org/a-kingdom-of-little-animals/.
3   In 1913, Marconi Transatlantic Wireless Telegraph's breathless report ... 'World Doctors Hail Ehrlich As Hero.' *New York Times*. https://www.nytimes.com/1913/08/09/archives/world-doctors-hail-ehrlich-as-hero-discoverer-of-salvarsan-tells.html.
4   Eric Lax recounts the story and reapportions ... Lax, E. *The Mold in Dr. Florey's Coat: The Story of the Penicillin Miracle.* New York: H. Holt, 2004, 1–336.
5   The need for antibiotics was recognized then ... Podolsky, S.H. *The Antibiotic Era: Reform, Resistance, and the Pursuit of a Rational Therapeutics.* Baltimore: Johns Hopkins University Press, 2015.
6   The *New York Times* celebrated its efficacy ... Laurence, William L. 'Science; Drug for Staph Widespread Germ Succumbs to a New Synthetic Penicillin.' *New York Times*, 12

March 1961. https://www.nytimes.com/1961/03/12/archives/science-drug-for-staph-widespread-germ-succumbs-to-a-new-synthetic.html.

7 **The findings of this year-long project** . . . Woodruff, H.B. Selman A. Waksman, Winner of the 1952 Nobel Prize for Physiology or Medicine. *Applied and Environmental Microbiology,* 80, no. 1, 2–8, 2014. https://journals.asm.org/doi/full/10.1128/aem.01143-13.

8 **In a seminal paper published in *Soil Science*** . . . Waksman, S.A. and R.L. Starkey. 'Partial Sterilization of Soil, Microbiological Activities and Soil Fertility: II.' *Soil Science,* 16, no. 4: 247–68, 1923.

9 **studies confirmed that streptomycin was safe** . . . Schatz, A., E. Bugle and S.A. Waksman. 'Streptomycin, a Substance Exhibiting Antibiotic Activity against Gram-Positive and Gram-Negative Bacteria.' *Proceedings of the Society for Experimental Biology and Medicine,* 55: 66–69, 1944.

10 **An editorial perspective in *The Lancet Infectious Diseases* in 2005** . . . Editorial. 'The Nobel Cause.' *The Lancet Infectious Diseases,* 5: 665, 2005.

11 **a commentary written by microbiologist Kim Lewis** . . . Lewis, K. 'Antibiotics: Recover the Lost Art of Drug Discovery.' *Nature,* 485: 439–40, 2012.

12 **In a 1963 article in the journal *Bacteriology Reviews*** . . . Watanabe, T. 'Infective Heredity of Multiple Drug Resistance in Bacteria.' *Bacteriological Review,* 27, no. 1: 87–115, 1963.

13 **In 1992, Stuart Levy, one of Watanabe's students** . . . Levy, S.B. *The Antibiotic Paradox: How the Misuse of Antibiotics Destroys Their Curative Power.* 1–296, 2002.

10. Drowning in Antibiotics

1 **The wastewater from the local treatment plant, responsible for processing** ... Fick, J. et al. 'Contamination of Surface, Ground, and Drinking Water from Pharmaceutical Production.' *Environmental Toxicology and Chemistry*, 28, no. 12: 2522–27, 2009.

2 **On an immediate level, this environmental contamination** ... Larsson, D.G.J. and C.F. Flach. 'Antibiotic Resistance in the Environment.' *Nature Reviews Microbiology*, 20: 257–69, 2022.

3 **Yet, a separate scientific study painted** ... Akhter, S. et al. 'Profiling of Antibiotic Residues in Surface Water of River Yamuna Stretch Passing through Delhi, India.' *Water* (Switzerland), 15, no. 3: 527, 2023.

4 **Water is also undoubtedly a primary source for the spread** ... Davies, J. and Dorothy Davis. 'Origins and Evolution of Antibiotic Resistance.' *Microbiology and Molecular Biology Reviews*, 74: 417–33, 2010.

5 **The WHO has spotlighted climate change** ... Adhanom, Tedros, Sultan Ahmed Al Jaber and Vanessa Kerry. 'We Must Fight One of the World's Biggest Health Threats – Climate Change.' World Health Organization. https://www.who.int/news-room/commentaries/detail/we-must-fight-one-of-the-world-s-biggest-health-threats-climate-change.

6 **In May 2018, a study published in *Nature Climate Change*** ... MacFadden, D.R. et al. 'Antibiotic Resistance Increases with Local Temperature.' *Nature Climate Change*, 8: 510–14, 2018.

7 **In August 2023, a study published in the *Lancet Planetary Health*** ... Zhou, Z. et al. 'Association Between Particulate Matter PM 2.5 Air Pollution and Clinical Antibiotic Resistance.' *The Lancet Planetary Health*, 7, no. 8: e649–e659, 2023.

11. Fat Animals and Antibiotics

1 **This story, which is expertly narrated by** . . . McKenna, M. *Plucked! The Truth About Chicken.* New York: Little, Brown, 2017.

2 **In 1950, upon the official revelation of Jukes's discovery** . . . Wellcome Trust. 'We Must Stop Squandering Our Precious Antibiotics.' https://wellcome.org/news/we-must-stop-squandering-our-precious-antibiotics.

3 **In a paper published in the *New England Journal of Medicine* in 1976** . . . Levy, S.B., G.B. FitzGerald and A.B. Macone. 'Changes in Intestinal Flora of Farm Personnel after Introduction of a Tetracycline-Supplemented Feed on a Farm.' *The New England Journal of Medicine*, 295: 583–88, 1976.

4 **In 1977, Donald Kennedy who was then** . . . Smith, Harrison. 'Stuart Levy, Microbiologist Who Sounded Alarm on . . .' *Washington Post*, 19 September 2019. https://www.washingtonpost.com/local/obituaries/stuart-levy-microbiologist-who-sounded-alarm-on-antibiotic-resistance-dies-at-80/2019/09/19/4011ea96-dae9-11e9-a688-303693fb4b0b_story.html.

5 **Today, we are caught in a web that has been spun from decades** . . . Van Boeckel, T.P. et al. 'Global Trends in Antimicrobial Use in Food Animals.' *Proceedings of the National Academy of Sciences of the United States of America*, 112, no. 18: 5649–54, 2015.

6 **In fact, it is estimated that over** . . . Mulchandani, R., et al. 'Global Trends in Antimicrobial Use in Food-Producing Animals: 2020 to 2030.' *PLOS Global Public Health*, 3, no. 2: e0001305, 2023.

7 **In 2016, all 193 member states of the United Nations** . . .

World Health Organization. 'At UN, Global Leaders Commit to Act on Antimicrobial Resistance.' https://www.who.int/news/item/21-09-2016-at-un-global-leaders-commit-to-act-on-antimicrobial-resistance.

8   **In 2018, a widely published investigative report . . .** The Bureau of Investigative Journalism. 'A Game of Chicken: How Indian Poultry Farming Is Creating Global Superbugs'. https://www.thebureauinvestigates.com/stories/2018-01-30/a-game-of-chicken-how-indian-poultry-farming-is-creating-global-superbugs.

12. A Market Failure

1   **However, as Scott Podolsky highlights . . .** Podolsky, S.H. *The Antibiotic Era: Reform, Resistance, and the Pursuit of a Rational Therapeutics*, 1–309. Baltimore: Johns Hopkins University Press, 2015.

2   **In 2022, a WHO report identified forty-six antibiotics and thirty-four non-traditional antibacterial treatments . . .** World Health Organization. *2021 Antibacterial Agents in Clinical and Preclinical Development: An Overview and Analysis*. World Health Organization, 2022.

3   **Regrettably, most other antibiotics and antibacterial drugs . . .** Butler, M.S. et al. 'Antibiotics in the Clinical Pipeline as of December 2022.' *Journal of Antibiotics*, 76: 431–73, 2023. Preprint at https://doi.org/10.1038/s41429-023-00629-8.

4   **Researchers often sift through thousands . . .** Shlaes, D.M. 'The Economic Conundrum for Antibacterial Drugs.' *Antimicrobial Agents and Chemotherapy*, 64, no. 1, 2020. Preprint at https://doi.org/10.1128/AAC.02057-19.

5   **Some estimates peg the costs . . .** Hall, William, Anthony

McDonnell and Jim O'Neill. *Superbugs: An Arms Race against Bacteria*, 246. Boston: Harvard University Press, 2018.

6   **Developing new drugs is a complex and costly...** Buckley, G.J. and G.H. Palmer (eds), *Combating Antimicrobial Resistance and Protecting the Miracle of Modern Medicine*. National Academies Press, 2022. DOI:10.17226/26350.

7   **A news article in the *Wall Street Journal* published...** Mosbergen, Dominique. 'The World Needs New Antibiotics. The Problem Is, No One Can Make Them Profitably.' *Wall Street Journal*, 26 September 2003. Available at: https://www.wsj.com/tech/biotech/antibiotics-drug-development-business-fda-aa5b4f00.

8   **The paradox of drug-pricing and the challenge it presents is summed up aptly...** Hall, William, Anthony McDonnell and Jim O'Neill. *Superbugs: An Arms Race against Bacteria*, 1–246. Boston: Harvard University Press, 2018

13. The Next Generation

1   **During the early days of antibiotic discovery...** Alam, K. et al. 'Streptomyces: The Biofactory of Secondary Metabolites.' *Frontiers in Microbiology*. 13: 2022. DOI: 10.3389/fmicb.2022.968053.

2   **They found a new antibiotic called teixobactin...** Ling, L.L. et al. 'A New Antibiotic Kills Pathogens Without Detectable Resistance.' *Nature*, 517: 455–59, 2015.

3   **In addition, it works through a two-step process...** Shukla, R. et al. 'Teixobactin Kills Bacteria by a Two-Pronged Attack on the Cell Envelope.' *Nature*, 608: 390–96, 2022.

4   **The team created fewer than a hundred...** Bugworks. 'Bugworks Research Announces the First in Human Phase

1 Study of BWC0977 for the Treatment of Critical Bacterial Infections.' Bugworks Research Announces the First in Human Phase 1 Study of BWC0977 for the Treatment of Critical Bacterial Infections, 8 November 2021. https://www.prnewswire.com/news-releases/bugworks-research-announces-the-first-in-human-phase-1-study-of-bwc0977-for-the-treatment-of-critical-bacterial-infections-301417408.html.

5 **Chemist Andrew Myers and his team at Harvard University**... Seiple, I.B. et al. 'A Platform for the Discovery of New Macrolide Antibiotics.' *Nature*, 533: 338–45, 2016.

6 **Myers' method is more direct**... Ledford, H. 'Hundreds of Antibiotics Built from Scratch.' *Nature*, 2016. DOI: 10.1038/nature.2016.19946.

7 **In a paper published in *Nature Chemical Biology***... Liu, G. et al. 'Deep Learning-Guided Discovery of an Antibiotic Targeting *Acinetobacter baumannii*.' *Nature Chemical Biology*, 19: 1342–50, 2023.

8 **Earlier, in 2020, the same researchers had shown**... Stokes, J.M. et al. 'A Deep Learning Approach to Antibiotic Discovery.' *Cell*, 180: 688–702, 2020.

9 **In December 2023, as I was finishing up writing this book**... Wong, F., et al. 'Discovery of a Structural Class of Antibiotics with Explainable Deep Learning.' *Nature*. https://doi.org/10.1038/s41586-023-06887-8.

14. Beyond Antibiotics

1 **Tom Patterson and Steffanie Strathdee never expected**... Strathdee, S. and Thomas Patterson. *The Perfect Predator: A Scientist's Race to Save Her Husband from a Deadly Superbug*. New York: Hachette Books, 2019, 1–352.

Notes

2   **Speaking later to the BBC, Strathdee recalled . . .** Lipman, N. Natasha. 'My Husband Squeezed My Hand to Say He Wanted to Live, Then I Found a Way to Save Him.' BBC News, 4 November 2019. https://www.bbc.com/news/stories-50221375.

3   **You can go to a pharmacy . . .** Parfitt, T. 'Georgia: An Unlikely Stronghold for Bacteriophage Therapy.' *The Lancet*, 365, no. 9478: 2166–67, 2005.

4   **Not everyone is convinced that . . .** Abedon, S.T. et al. 'Bacteriophage Prehistory.' *Bacteriophage* 1, no. 3: 174–78, 2011.

5   **Its versatility, ranging from natural to genetically engineered . . .** Strathdee, S.A. et al. 'Phage Therapy: From Biological Mechanisms to Future Directions.' *Cell*, 186, no. 1: 17–31, 2023.

6   **Perhaps the greatest limitation to phage therapy . . .** Fabijan, A.P. et al. 'Translating Phage Therapy into the Clinic: Recent Accomplishments but Continuing Challenges.' *PLoS Biology*, 21, no. 5: e3002119, 2023.

7   **A landmark study published in 2023 in the *BMJ Global Health* . . .** Kim, C. et al. 'Global and Regional Burden of Attributable and Associated Bacterial Antimicrobial Resistance Avertable by Vaccination.' *BMJ Global Health*, 8, no. 7: e011341, 2023.

8   **In general, there are more vaccines . . .** Micoli, F. et al. 'The Role of Vaccines in Combatting Antimicrobial Resistance.' *Nature Reviews Microbiology*, 19: 287–302, 2021. Preprint at https://doi.org/10.1038/s41579-020-00506-3.

9   **One of the front-line defenders of this system . . .** Fjell, C.D. et al. 'Designing Antimicrobial Peptides: Form Follows Function.' *Nature Reviews Drug Discovery*, 11: 37–51, 2012. Preprint at https://doi.org/10.1038/nrd3591.

10 **Two modern concepts in gut health** . . . Wolter, M. et al. 'Leveraging Diet to Engineer the Gut Microbiome.' *Nature Reviews Gastroenterology & Hepatology*, 18: 885–902, 2021. Preprint at https://doi.org/10.1038/s41575-021-00512-7.

11 **In the case of *Clostridioides difficile* infections** . . . Sorbara, M. T. and E.G. Pamer. 'Microbiome-based Therapeutics.' *Nature Reviews Microbiology*, 20: 365–80, 2022.

15. The Hidden Pandemic

1 **Between 2000 and 2015** . . . Klein, E.Y. et al. 'Global Increase and Geographic Convergence in Antibiotic Consumption between 2000 and 2015.' *Proceedings of the National Academy of Sciences of the United States of America*, 115, no. 15: E3463–E3470, 2018.

2 **Globally, over 210,000 infant deaths** . . . Jasovský, D. et al. 'Antimicrobial Resistance – A Threat to the World's Sustainable Development.' *Upsala Journal of Medical Sciences*, 121, no. 3: 159–64, 2016.

3 **A 2023 study of fifty-nine low- and medium-income countries** . . . Hossain, M.S. et al. 'Antibiotic Prescription from Qualified Sources for Children with Fever/Cough.' *EClinicalMedicine*, 61: 2023. DOI: 10.1016/j.eclinm.2023.102055.

4 **Today, despite guidelines recommending shorter treatment periods** . . . Spellberg, B. 'The Maturing Antibiotic Mantra: "Shorter Is Still Better."' *Journal of Hospital Medicine*, 13, no. 5: 361–62, 2018.

Acknowledgements

First and foremost, my heartfelt gratitude goes to my family, whose patience and steadfast support have been the pillars of my strength. To Arhan, my most enthusiastic cheerleader and most rigorous critic – your curiosity and inquisitiveness signal a promising future in science (or any field you choose to embrace). I also extend my thanks to my mother-in-law, Anjali Panigrahi. Though she did not live to see the publication of this book, I know she would have been immensely proud.

To my publisher, Chiki Sarkar, for seeing potential in my thoughts and reaching out – this book wouldn't exist without your faith. The journey of writing is often solitary but knowing that someone believes in your vision makes every challenging step worthwhile.

My editor, Devangshu Datta, your patience has been extraordinary, especially when I veered off our agreed deadlines. Your commitment to making this work the best it could possibly be never wavered, even when mine did. For that, I am truly grateful.

Acknowledgements

A special nod to Sakshi Pandit and Parag Sahasrabudhe for critiquing the manuscript. Your insights were invaluable in ensuring the accuracy and engagement of this book.

While I've had the privilege of guidance and support from many, it is essential to clarify that the opinions expressed within these pages, as well as any inadvertent errors, are entirely my own. In particular, the viewpoints or oversights present in this book should not be attributed to my employer.

Please note that the content provided in this book is for informational purposes only and is not intended as medical advice. The information contained here should not be used as a substitute for professional diagnoses or treatment. Always seek the advice of your physician or other qualified health providers with any questions you may have regarding a medical condition.

To everyone else who played a part in the realization of this project – your contributions are deeply cherished. To all of you who stood by me during this process, heartfelt thanks!